MOSBY'S

MASSAGE
THERAPY
REVIEW

MOSBY'S

MASSAGE THERAPY REVIEW

SANDY FRITZ, MS

Founder, Owner, Director, and Head Instructor
Health Enrichment Center
School of Therapeutic Massage and Bodywork
Lapeer, Michigan

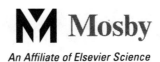 Mosby

An Affiliate of Elsevier Science

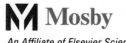

An Affiliate of Elsevier Science

Publishing Director: John A. Schrefer
Associate Editor: Kellie F. White
Developmental Editor: Jennifer L. Watrous
Project Manager: Peggy Fagen
Designer: Renée Duenow

Mosby, Inc.
An Affiliate of Elsevier Science
11830 Westline Industrial Drive
St. Louis, Missouri 63146

Printed in the United States of America

International Standard Book Number 0-323-01738-X

03 04 05 FG/EB 9 8 7 6 5 4 3 2

Dedicated to the Health Enrichment Center, Inc.,
Graduating Class, August 2001

Special thanks to M. James Grosenbach, EdD,
for his special efforts in reading and assisting in the development
of valid question structure and the design of the text.

Introduction

This study guide has been created to support the therapeutic massage student and graduate through a review process preparing for various educational evaluations such as midterm and final exams, and local, state, and national licensing or certification exams. The questions are based on *Mosby's Basic Science for Soft Tissue and Movement Therapies* and *Mosby's Fundamentals of Therapeutic Massage*, ed. 2.

Information presented in most educational curriculums and information required to function as a massage professional can be divided into four areas. These categories form the basis of most licensing and certifying examinations. The four categories are:
- Human Anatomy, Physiology, and Kinesiology
- Clinical Pathology and Indications and Contraindications for Massage Application
- Massage Therapy and Bodywork
- Professional Standards, Ethics, and Business Practices

Four Areas of Preparation

1. Human Anatomy, Physiology, and Kinesiology
This general education prepares the student to understand the benefits of massage and lays the foundation for the following area.

2. Clinical Pathology and Indications and Contraindications for Massage Application
Human anatomy, physiology, kinesiology, clinical pathology, and indications and contraindications for massage application cover half of the content on most exams. The focus is to provide sufficient information to support safe and beneficial professional practice.

Usually these two categories are most effectively studied in an integrated format. For example, discussion of the anatomy of the nervous system leads to understanding the functions of the nervous system. Subsequently, understanding how massage affects the nervous system leads to identification of indications for massage and the nervous system, pathology of the nervous system, and contraindications for applications of massage, including cautions for use of massage when pathologic conditions are present.

Many find the sciences a more difficult study area. The terminology can seem overwhelming—almost like learning another language. If we can agree that the various methods and theoretical base of the many different bodywork modalities provide diversity, then the sciences provide commonality. The human body in structure and function remains consistent; therefore, it makes sense that an understanding of the sciences is essential and relevant to massage.

Non-Western science content is primarily focused on traditional Chinese medicine but also covers other energy systems such as Shiatsu, Polarity therapy, and Ayurveda.

3. Massage Therapy and Bodywork: Theory and Application
Competency in this area indicates that the massage professional is able to appropriately apply methods in a safe and beneficial way. There is a commonality in most bodywork approaches. The content in this area covers methods used to obtain a database about the client and proper methods usage.

In addition to therapeutic massage, general knowledge about complementary bodywork modalities such as hydrotherapy, Asian theory, and applications such as acupressure, trigger points, and connective tissue massage is often measured.

4. Professional Ethics and Business Practices
The professional standards, ethics, and business practices area develops the professional abilities needed to conduct oneself in a manner that reflects decision making to support ethical standards and sound business practices.

Sample Questions in Relation to the Four Areas of Study

On an exam these four categories are addressed specifically within a test question or the content is mixed to develop combination test questions. For example, a pure science question may appear as follows: "The largest of the fontanels in the infant skull is _____?" An example of a question combining content may appear as follows: "During infant massage it is important to apply only light pressure to the anterior fontanel for which of the following reasons?"

ANALYZING THE QUESTION

A good multiple-choice question presents sufficient facts so that the correct answer can be identified. The four possible answers need to be analyzed based on the facts presented in the question and your knowledge in order to determine the best correct answer. All possible answers should be plausible and the incorrect answers should not be evident. Analyzing the possible answers requires a comprehensive factual base provided during your education and found in the textbooks so that wrong answers can be eliminated and the correct answer identified and justified.

In this review guide each sample question embodies a chunk of essential knowledge and is a representation of how that knowledge is often addressed in a multiple-choice exam. Each of the four possible answers also identifies important information. When using the questions to study for an exam, the information in all of the possible answers, the one correct answer, and the three incorrect answers should be identified in the textbooks. The correct answer should clearly stand out and the reasons why incorrect answers are false should be apparent. Many of the questions are framed in mini case studies, since this is a more relevant format for practitioners as they use the information in context of the client population they serve.

TYPES OF MULTIPLE-CHOICE QUESTIONS

There are three basic types of multiple-choice questions: factual recall and comprehension, application and concept identification, and clinical reasoning and synthesis. Examples of the three types of questions follow.

1. Factual Recall and Comprehension

The information necessary to answer this type of question can be found in various textbooks in the form of descriptions and definitions. Memorization of data is a method that can be used to prepare to answer these types of questions. An example of this type of question is:

Which bone makes up the heel of the foot?

a. Navicular
b. Calcaneus
c. Hamate
d. Xyphoid

The answer is b.

2. Application and Concept Identification

This type of question requires that you understand the language posed in the question or be able to identify simple concepts and patterns. In addition, this type of question measures one's ability to understand language as it relates to contextual frameworks. Application and concept identification questions also address concrete information that can be described in terms, definitions, rules, laws, and other forms of structure. This information can be found directly in the textbooks. An example of this type of question is:

Which method would be most appropriate if the client desires to remain passive during the massage?

a. Pulsed muscle energy
b. Reciprocal inhibition
c. Approximation
d. Postisometric relaxation

The answer is c.

3. Clinical Reasoning/Synthesis

Clinical reasoning/synthesis questions require you to analyze information and make appropriate professional decisions. Identifying the answer to this type of question requires that the information be used in a contextual manner. The case study scenario is a common approach to this question design. The answer is not found directly in any textbook; only the language and concepts would be in the textbooks. An example of this type of question is:

A client is taking an aspirin for osteoarthritis of the left knee. What precautions are needed for massage intervention?

a. Avoid any type of massage to the affected knee.
b. Avoid the use of compression above and below the knee.
c. Reduce pressure level around the knee only.
d. Monitor pressure levels of the massage to reduce potential bruising.

The answer is d.

Make the Textbooks Work For You

The questions in the first two sections of this review guide are presented sequentially, chapter by chapter, as described in *Mosby's Basic Science for Soft Tissue and Movement Therapies* and *Mosby's Fundamentals of Therapeutic Massage*, ed. 2. The answers and rationales are located at the end of each chapter. Other textbooks can be used as resources as well by looking up the content in the index. In an actual exam, the content will be mixed up. Section III provides questions that overlap knowledge with application, theory, ethics, and sciences, since this represents how knowledge acquired for formal massage training and self-study is used in professional practice. The labeling exercises in Section IV, while not found on an exam, are an effective study tool.

The Mosby textbooks are designed as interactive work texts, making them excellent for self-study. Space is provided within the text for completion of activities, exercises, and workbook sections. If you resist writing in the book, do the exercises on pages copied from the textbooks.

Each chapter covers a large piece of knowledge. Chapter objectives reflect suggested competencies for the content. The chapters are relatively large, so each chapter is divided into sections. These sections also have objectives. Subheadings divide sections into smaller bits of information that can be processed in about 15 minutes of reading. This supports most people's sustained attention span.

An activity or exercise corresponds with the various subheadings. For memory retention, it is important for the information to be manipulated in some way. Various strategies are used to support this information retention, such as paraphrasing, metaphors, drawings, practical applications, relationship to personal experiences, and movement. Use these activities and exercises as points of study. Each chapter ends with a workbook section. The workbook is designed to summarize the chapter. At the end of the workbook is an answer key. The answer key is like a chapter summary (e.g., Cliff Notes). There is also some sort of problem-solving activity in each workbook section. These take the form of professional application exercises, problem-solving activities, or research for further study. This type of activity helps develop clinical reasoning skills necessary to successfully address the clinical reasoning synthesis-type exam questions. After you have studied the chapter in the textbook, then challenge yourself with the questions in this study guide that relate to the chapter content.

Completing all of the interactive exercises, activities, and self-study using this study guide should be adequate preparation for educational exams and the licensing and certification exams currently being used. Recommended textbook lists for exam preparation are usually available from those that administer the various exams. It is prudent to obtain these lists and compare the information to be confidently prepared for the challenge of an exam.

Accompanying this review guide is a CD-ROM. These are two testing features available on this CD to aid in studying for massage exams. The "Tutorial" mode serves questions by category and provides instant feedback including rationales. The "Test" mode randomly serves questions and allows for review after a test has been completed.

Many test questions and answers from Sections I and II in the review guide are included. While questions in the review guide are arranged by content area, the CD randomizes the questions, which provides a more realistic representation of electronic exams. Each practice exam consists of 200 questions. A scoring matrix is provided after each and presents the overall number of attempted and correct questions, as well as the percentage of correct answers. The matrix also provides information regarding the four categories emphasized in the review guide (Human Anatomy, Physiology, and Kinesiology; Pathology and Condition Recognition; Massage Therapy and Bodywork; and Standards, Ethics, and Business Practice) and indicating the student's score in each category. Following the categories is a breakdown of the chapters from the review guide, again showing the number of attempted questions, the number of correct answers, and the percentage of correct answers.

Once the user has reviewed the scoring matrix, the "Tutorial" mode can be used to emphasize areas of weakness that have been identified. For example, if a low percentage was scored in Pathology and Condition Recognition, the user can bring up the tutorial and practice questions in that category only.

Recommendations for Studying For An Exam

1. Relax. Anxiety interferes with the ability to integrate and recall information.
2. Have fun and be silly. Things learned with laughter are more easily retained.
3. Study in short bursts. Thirty minutes at a time is ideal.
4. Generally read a chapter and then study one small section at a time.
5. Know the meaning of any words displayed in key terms lists, in bold or italics print, and in the glossary and be able to use the words correctly in a sentence.

6. Study the illustrations and diagrams, paying attention to the labeling.
7. Manipulate the information. The interactive exercises and workbook segments of *Mosby's Fundamentals of Therapeutic Massage,* ed. 2, and *Mosby's Basic Science for Soft Tissue and Movement Therapies* are designed to integrate information from short-term to long-term memory. Other textbooks often offer similar features.
8. Seek to understand the information. Do not anticipate the test. Paraphrase and reword the information presented in the text.
9. Use the questions in this study guide as a study strategy. The questions are organized sequentially chapter by chapter in each of the textbooks. Write your own exam questions. The most difficult task is developing plausible wrong answers. (Use the questions in this book as examples.)
10. Work together in study groups by either sharing information, by taking turns "teaching," or by taking each other's tests from the questions you wrote.

Recommendations for Taking an Exam

1. Get plenty of rest before the exam.
2. Arrive at the exam location in plenty of time to settle into the environment.
3. Ask questions about the exam process so that you clearly understand how to take the exam.
4. Acknowledge that you are nervous, relax as much as you can, and put the exam in perspective. The worst that can happen is that you might not pass. This only means more study and another attempt. The best that can happen is that you pass.
5. Begin at the beginning of the exam and answer questions sequentially.
6. If the answer to a question is not apparent to you, mark the question and return to it after the exam

is completed. Often other questions on the exam will provide information to help you answer the question you skipped over.
7. When the exam is finished, go back and answer the skipped questions. If you still do not know the answer, guess and let intuition work. Do not leave a space blank. A blank is wrong and a guess is possible.
8. Do not second-guess your answers. Only change an answer if you are sure that you were wrong with your first choice.
9. Review the exam to make sure you answered all the questions and that basic information such as your name, etc. is completed.
10. Turn in the exam as instructed and breathe. It is over—no sense worrying—remember perspective—go do something fun.

The questions found in this guide will not appear on any exam. Instead, they are written to reflect both the type of questions encountered on educational and certification and licensing exams and as a sequential study through the sciences, theory, business, and ethics of the practice of therapeutic massage and related bodywork modalities. The questions have been carefully thought out so that if you study both the question and all the possible answers (correct and incorrect), you should have the factual knowledge and the critical thinking skills to confidently approach an exam. Just because you can answer all the questions in this study guide does not mean that you will pass an exam. It is the ability to be confident in one's knowledge and problem-solving skills that will assure success, not memorization of the questions and answers in this book or any other textbook or study guide.

Success to you!

Sandy Fritz

Contents

S E C T I O N   I I I

S E C T I O N   I V

A P P E N D I C E S

MOSBY'S
MASSAGE THERAPY REVIEW

I

CHAPTER

1

The Body as a Whole

Questions

1. Adenosine triphosphate (ATP) releases energy in muscles by what process? *(metabolism)*

   a. Mitosis
   b. Interphase
   c. Catabolism *(5½) - break down*
   d. Anabolism *- build up*

2. The substance between cell tissues made up of ground substance and fibers is called _____.

   a. Matrix
   b. Nucleic acids
   c. Basement membrane
   d. Meiosis

3. In relation to anatomy and physiology, the phrase "structure and function" involves _____.

   a. Gross anatomy translates to regional anatomy
   b. Anatomy guides physiology and is modified by function
   c. Systemic physiology involves organizational anatomy
   d. Duality of wholeness represented in catabolism and anabolism

4. The complementary relationship of opposites is described by _____.

   a. Organ and system organization
   b. Responsiveness and metabolism
   c. Yin and yang
   d. Qi and shen

5. How do we use physiology in the application of massage?

   a. Location of structures to be manipulated
   b. Specific positioning of the client for assessment
   c. Decision making relating to projected outcomes
   d. Directional communication in charting

6. Characteristics of life involve _____.

   a. Physiology
   b. Yin
   c. Anatomy
   d. Tissue

7. The chemical reaction that occurs in cells to effect transformation, production, or consumption of energy is _____.

   a. Absorption
   b. Digestion
   c. Responsiveness
   d. Metabolism

8. The process of homeostasis is a logical well-coordinated pattern of balance. When balance is disrupted patterns of dysfunction occur. Often both homeostasis and disease begin at what level of body organization?

   a. Chemical
   b. Cellular
   c. Tissue
   d. Organ

9. *The concept of yang as compared to atomic structure is _____.*

    a. Nucleus
    b. Protons
    c. Electrons
    d. Neutrons

10. *Atomic bonding to form molecules occurs because of the action among _____.*

    a. Nuclei
    b. Protons
    c. Electrons
    d. Neutrons

11. *The most stable of atomic bonds is the _____.*

    a. Ionic bond
    b. Covalent bond
    c. Polar covalent bond
    d. Catabolic bond

12. *Which type of atomic bond holds together DNA?*

    a. Ionic bond
    b. Covalent bond
    c. Polar covalent bond
    d. Catabolic bond

13. *When chemical bonds are broken and new ones formed, what has occurred?*

    a. Mitochondrial reactivity
    b. Hydrolysis response
    c. Conductivity interaction
    d. Chemical reaction

14. *The physiologic process that converts food and air into energy is called _____.*

    a. Metabolism
    b. Homeostasis
    c. Anabolism
    d. Dehydration

15. *Massage creates chemical reactions in what way?*

    a. Generates a stimulus
    b. Encourages interphase
    c. Supports hypertrophy
    d. Disrupts differentiation

16. *Which of the following chemical reactions uses energy when complex compounds are formed?*

    a. Anabolism
    b. Metabolism
    c. Catabolism
    d. Mitosis

17. *The study of chemical actions in the body is of what importance to the massage professional?*

    a. Charting is dependent upon these interactions
    b. Many massage benefits are derived from chemical reactions
    c. Validation of subtle energy will be atomic
    d. Chemical reactions are responsible for all pathology

18. *Which of the following organelles is involved in manufacture of proteins?*

    a. Endoplasmic reticulum
    b. Mitochondria
    c. Lysosomes
    d. Ribosomes

19. *The most abundant component in cells is _____.*

    a. Water
    b. Protein
    c. Lipids
    d. Carbohydrates

20. *Cell division is the reproductive process of cells called _____.*

    a. Interphase
    b. Mitosis
    c. Cytosol
    d. Catabolism

21. When a cell is able to perform a specialized function, the structure of the cell is modified. This is called _____.

    a. Hypertrophy
    b. Atrophy
    c. Differentiation
    d. Meiosis

22. Basement membrane connects epithelial tissue to _____.

    a. Muscle tissue
    b. Nervous tissue
    c. Neutrophil tissue
    d. Connective tissue

23. Which of the following is considered a cutaneous membrane?

    a. Skin
    b. Mucous membrane
    c. Serous membrane
    d. Collagen

24. Which of the following membranes line cavities not open to the external environments and many organs?

    a. Basement membranes *(epit)*
    b. Mucous membranes
    c. Serous membranes
    d. Cutaneous membranes *(skin)*

25. Which of the following tissues are the most abundant in the body?

    a. Epithelial tissue
    b. Connective tissue
    c. Muscle tissue
    d. Nervous tissue

26. Specialization of connective tissue is focused to _____.

    a. Support
    b. Contractility
    c. Excitability
    d. Hypertrophy

27. The diverse forms of connective tissue are attributed to _____.

    a. Properties of cells and composition of matrix
    b. Extensive distribution of blood vessels
    c. The distribution of chondroblasts in the matrix
    d. The collagen formation of ground substance

28. The connective tissue type with the most blood flow is _____.

    a. Cartilage
    b. Dense irregular
    c. Areolar
    d. Dense regular

29. The type of connective tissue most often found in ligaments and tendons is _____.

    a. Dense regular
    b. Dense irregular
    c. Areolar
    d. Adipose

30. Which following cell type is found in the connective tissue matrix that secretes bone?

    a. Fibroblast
    b. Chondroblast
    c. Osteoblast
    d. Hemocytoblast

31. Which of the following cartilage types is most likely to be damaged from wear and tear of the hip or knee joint?

    a. Hyaline cartilage
    b. Fibrocartilage
    c. Elastic cartilage
    d. Reticular cartilage

32. *Massage methods applied to the connective tissue have benefit because of its thixotropic properties. This means _____.*

    a. Massage stimulates mast cells to release histamine to reduce inflammation
    b. Massage separates the desmosomes and gap junctions to allow flexibility
    c. Massage increases the secretion of synovial fluid to increase joint mobility
    d. Massage acts to agitate ground substance and encourages a softer, more pliable tissue texture

33. *What property of collagen may make it viable in the generation of body energy?*

    a. Resistance to deformation
    b. Piezoelectric aspects
    c. Colloid formation
    d. Macrophagic activity

34. *The Oriental healing theory of the Law of Five Elements relates best to _____.*

    a. Muscle tissue structures
    b. Nervous tissue structures
    c. Organs
    d. Prana

35. *Which of the following would be considered yin?*

    a. Heart
    b. Stomach
    c. Body systems
    d. Qi

Answers and Discussion

1. **c**
Factual recall
Rationale: ATP is a compound that stores energy in muscle. This energy is released during the chemical process of catabolism.

2. **a**
Factual recall
Rationale: The question is the definition of matrix.

3. **b**
Application and concept identification
Rationale: Anatomy is the study of the structure of the body and physiology is the study of the function of the body. This question asks for the relationship of the two.

4. **c**
Factual recall
Rationale: This question is asking for a definition of Oriental terminology, specifically yin and yang.

5. **c**
Application and concept identification
Rationale: The question asks for an application of the study of physiology to massage and bodywork. Most benefits from massage are the result of physiologic changes. The potential of these changes is a determinate of what will be the outcome of the massage.

6. **a**
Application and concept identification
Rationale: The question is asking for the relationship between two concepts that define life. While anatomy can be studied on cadavers, physiology is apparent when life is manifested.

7. **d**
Factual recall
Rationale: The question is a definition of metabolism.

8. **a**
Application and concept identification
Rationale: The question asks for an understanding of homeostasis and the relationship to the development of disease. The chemical level of the organizational structure of the body is often where homeostasis begins to break down and disease begins.

9. **b**
Application and concept identification
Rationale: Yang is considered positive energy flow and protons are the positively charged particles in an atom.

10. **c**
Factual recall
Rationale: The question describes a function of electrons.

11. **b**
Factual recall
Rationale: Ionic, covalent, and polar covalent are types of atomic bonds. Catabolic bond does not exist, so this is an incorrect word usage. Of the three, the covalent bond is most stable.

12. **c**
Application and concept identification
Rationale: DNA represents a type of molecule formed by a type of atomic bond. DNA is formed by polar covalent bonds.

13. **d**
Factual recall
Rationale: The question is the definition of a chemical reaction.

14. **a**
Factual recall
Rationale: The question is a definition of metabolism.

15. **a**
Application and concept identification
Rationale: The question asks for the interaction between the physiologic response to massage as a stimulus to chemical reactions.

16. **a**
Factual recall
Rationale: The question is the definition of anabolism.

17. **b**
Application and concept identification
Rationale: The question asks why the massage professional needs to understand chemical actions. The best answer is related to understanding the benefit of massage.

18. **d**
Factual recall
Rationale: The question describes an organelle function. Ribosomes manufacture proteins. An understanding of all organelle function is necessary to identify the correct answer.

19. **a**
Factual recall
Rationale: Of the four listed components that make up cells, water is the most abundant.

20. **b**
Factual recall
Rationale: Mitosis is the reproductive process of cells.

21. **c**
Factual recall
Rationale: The question is the definition of differentiation.

22. **d**
Factual recall
Rationale: The question describes a function of basement membrane.

23. **a**
Factual recall
Rationale: Skin is the largest cutaneous membrane.

24. **c**
Factual recall
Rationale: The question is the definition of serous membranes.

25. **b**
Factual recall
Rationale: Of the four tissue types, connective tissue is the most abundant in the body.

26. **a**
Factual recall
Rationale: Support is a major function of connective tissue.

27. **a**
Application and concept identification
Rationale: The only answer provided that correctly described connective tissue is related to the properties of the cells and composition of the matrix. The other three answers incorrectly describe connective tissue.

28. **c**
Factual recall
Rationale: Areolar connective tissue has a high vascularity, unlike the other types mentioned, which have limited blood flow.

29. **a**
Factual recall
Rationale: The question describes the location of dense regular connective tissue.

30. **c**
Factual recall
Rationale: The question is the definition of an osteoblast.

31. **a**
Application and concept identification
Rationale: The question asks for the relationship between a type of cartilage and the function of a joint. Hyaline cartilage is found at the ends of bones in synovial joints such as the hip and knee and is subject to damage from repetitive movement.

32. **d**
Application and concept identification
Rationale: The question asks for the relationship between a massage application and a physiologic outcome of connective tissue. It is necessary to understand the terminology in both the question and the answers to identify the correct answer. The incorrect answers describe wrong physiologic processes or do not address the facts of the question. The only correct response is answer d.

33. **b**
Factual recall
Rationale: Deforming collagen creates a piezoelectric electric current.

34. **c**
Application and concept identification
Rationale: The Law of Five Elements is most directly correlated with the organs. Muscle and nerve tissue is too limited an answer, and prana is a term used to describe life energy.

35. **a**
Factual recall
Rationale: Understanding both terminology and definition of yin organ functions is necessary to identify the heart with yin.

2

Mechanisms of Health and Disease

Questions

1. The common relationship between yin/yang, the five element theory, and Ayurvedic dosha is _____.

   a. Entrainment
   b. Somatic
   c. Homeostasis
   d. Etiology

2. Ayurvedic theory classifies physiologic functions by _____.

   a. Elements
   b. Visceral function
   c. Feedback
   d. Doshas

3. Which of the following represent principles of movement?

   a. Pitta
   b. Vata
   c. Kapha
   d. Ether

4. Feedback is an essential aspect of homeostasis because of _____.

   a. Afferent discharge
   b. Effector response
   c. Information exchange
   d. Efferent signaling

5. Any stimulus that disrupts internal homeostasis is _____.

   a. Consciousness
   b. Negative feedback
   c. Stress
   d. Pathology

6. A sensor mechanism, integration/control center, and effector mechanism are all part of a _____.

   a. Stress response
   b. Postisometric relaxation
   c. Stimulus response
   d. Feedback loop

7. Feedback that reverses the original stimulus, stabilizing physiologic function, is _____.

   a. Positive feedback
   b. Negative feedback
   c. Stimulus response feedback
   d. Regulatory response

8. Massage is part of a feedback loop in the _____.

   a. Controlled condition
   b. Control center
   c. Response
   d. Stress stimulus

9. *Many benefits of massage are a result of _____.*

    a. Nonspecific stress stimulus that encourages feedback response to more optimum function
    b. Precise application of selected stimulus creating positive feedback
    c. Positive feedback response to return function to homeostasis
    d. Afferent transmission to the sensory mechanism with the disrupted homeostasis reduced by the control center

10. *Biologic rhythms are maintained by _____.*

    a. Circadian patterns
    b. Ultradian patterns
    c. Negative feedback
    d. Positive feedback

11. *Relaxed mood states are experienced by people when _____.*

    a. Biologic rhythms are entrained to sympathetic patterns
    b. Biologic rhythms are oscillated independently
    c. Biologic rhythms are entrained to the chakra system
    d. Biologic rhythms are entrained to parasympathetic patterns

12. *Relaxed ordered entrainment is produced by massage in response to _____.*

    a. The practitioner's direct application of methods
    b. The practitioner's calm presence and rhythmic application
    c. The practitioner's emotional state
    d. The practitioner's specific choice of methods that address the chakra system

13. *Relaxation methods that focus on breathing produce entrainment because _____.*

    a. Cortisol increases during parasympathetic response.
    b. Respiration rate is a major biologic oscillator
    c. Sympathetic mechanisms are generated
    d. Baroreceptors are inhibited

14. *An interesting similarity between the traditional chakra system and biologic oscillators is _____.*

    a. Rhythm patterns
    b. Vibratory rate
    c. Shared location
    d. Size comparison

15. *Evidence of a healthy state includes _____.*

    a. Adaptive capacity to stress
    b. Strain in response to stress
    c. Susceptibility to bacterial infection
    d. Stress exceeds adaptive capacity

16. *A massage professional needs an understanding of disease processes. This study of disease processes is called _____.*

    a. Pathogenesis
    b. Pathology
    c. Epidemiology
    d. Pharmacology

17. *A group of signs and symptoms that identify a pathologic condition linked to a common cause is called a/n _____.*

    a. Disease
    b. Diagnosis
    c. Etiology
    d. Syndrome

18. *A disease with a vague onset that develops slowly and remains active for a long period of time is considered _____.*

    a. Acute
    b. Communicable
    c. Chronic
    d. Idiopathic

19. *Susceptibility to the disruption of homeostasis extensive enough to cause disease could be due to which of the following factors?*

    a. Hyperplasia
    b. Malnutrition
    c. Antineoplastics
    d. Pathogenesis

20. *Pathogenic organisms are considered to be* _____.

    a. Parasites
    b. Chemical agents
    c. Allergy
    d. Neoplasm

21. *A neoplasm resulting from hyperplasia that is contained and encapsulated is considered* _____.

    a. Acute
    b. Chronic
    c. Benign
    d. Malignant

22. *Cancer cells' reproduction of undifferentiated cells without boundary recognition is called* _____.

    a. Replacement
    b. Carcinogens
    c. Metastasis
    d. Anaplasia

23. *Heat, redness, swelling, and pain are signs of* _____.

    a. Cancer
    b. Degeneration
    c. Counterirritation
    d. Inflammation

24. *Inflammatory exudate that accumulates during an inflammatory process* _____.

    a. Reduces swelling
    b. Dilutes irritants
    c. Inhibits tissue repair
    d. Causes the release of mediators of inflammation

25. *An inflammatory mediator that dilates blood vessels is* _____.

    a. Histamine
    b. Prostaglandins
    c. Inflammatory exudates
    d. Neutrophils

26. *The purpose of increased tissue fluid volume during inflammation is* _____

    a. To allow parenchymal cells to regenerate the area of injury
    b. To allow immune cells to travel quickly to destroy pathogens
    c. To support the activity of labile cells during tissue repair
    d. To increase the activity of histamine and kinins during tissue repair

27. *Tissue repair for regeneration of functional cells is accomplished by* _____.

    a. Stromal cells
    b. Labile cells
    c. Parenchymal cells
    d. Fibrin cells

28. *Tissue repair that results in a scar is called* _____.

    a. Stroma
    b. Replacement
    c. Regeneration
    d. Idiopathic

29. *A major component of scar tissue is* _____.

    a. Epidermis
    b. Epithelium
    c. Fibroblasts
    d. Collagen

30. *Inflammation that persists beyond beneficial healing is considered an inflammatory disease. This chronic form of inflammation may be helped with what form of massage?*

    a. Extensive application of deep transverse friction
    b. Light surface stroking
    c. Controlled use of friction, stretching, and pulling
    d. Brisk beating and pounding

---

31. *Systemic inflammatory responses and fibromyalgia are _____.*
    a. Indicated for massage that causes inflammation
    b. Indicated for massage that involves extensive stretching and pulling techniques
    c. Contraindicated for massage that causes inflammation
    d. Contraindicated for massage only in the area of the joints

32. *Genetics, age, lifestyles, stress, environment, and preexisting conditions are _____.*
    a. Determinates of immune hypersensitivity
    b. Predisposing risk factors for development of disease
    c. Potential distribution routes for pathogens
    d. Warning signs of cancer

33. *The number one complaint of people to their health care professional is _____.*
    a. Decreased circulation
    b. Joint stiffness
    c. Breathing difficulties
    d. Pain

34. *Potential tissue damage is signaled by _____.*
    a. Pain
    b. Inflammation
    c. Steroids
    d. Moxibustion

35. *The sensory mechanisms for pain are called _____.*
    a. Intractable
    b. Hyperalgesia
    c. Nociceptors
    d. Bradykinin

36. *Pain that is poorly localized, nauseating, and associated with sweating and blood pressure changes is _____.*
    a. Superficial somatic pain
    b. Burning pain
    c. Aching pain
    d. Deep pain

37. *Pain that may be a symptom of an organ disorder is _____.*
    a. Superficial somatic pain
    b. Burning pain
    c. Aching pain
    d. Deep pain

38. *Pain that arises from stimulation of receptors in the skin or from stimulation of receptors in skeletal muscles, joints, tendons, and fascia is called _____.*
    a. Visceral pain
    b. Phantom pain
    c. Somatic pain
    d. Referred pain

39. *A massage application that creates superficial somatic pain that blocks transmission of deep somatic or visceral pain is called _____.*
    a. Counterirritation
    b. Pain-spasm-pain cycle
    c. Reflex contraction
    d. Cutaneous stimulation

40. *When pain is felt in a surface area away from the stimulated receptors, particularly in organs, it is called _____.*
    a. Visceral pain
    b. Phantom pain
    c. Somatic pain
    d. Referred pain

41. *A client comes to you complaining of an aching pain just under the ribs right of the midline, under the right scapula, and in the right neck and shoulder area. The pain has been occurring on a more frequent basis and is now almost constant. The referred pain pattern might indicate problems with what organ?*

    a. Bladder
    b. Kidney
    c. Stomach
    d. Gallbladder

42. *A client's low back pain returns within 3 hours of receiving massage. What organ may be the cause of referred back pain?*

    a. Bladder
    b. Kidney
    c. Stomach
    d. Gallbladder

43. *A massage client does not provide effective feedback about the amount of pressure requested for massage. The client asks for very deep pressure. As the massage professional you keep asking if the pressure is causing pain and the client says no. It seems that any deeper pressure may cause bruising and other tissue damage. This client may be exhibiting _____.*

    a. Counterirritation
    b. Reduced influence of beta-endorphins
    c. High pain tolerance
    d. Hyperstimulation analgesia

44. *Massage used as a pain management strategy is a form of _____.*

    a. Stimulus-induced analgesia
    b. Acupuncture
    c. Dermatomal inhibition
    d. Prostaglandin stimulation

45. *Aspirin is used in pain management since its effects include _____.*

    a. Increased inflammation
    b. Inhibiting enkephalins
    c. Inhibiting prostaglandins
    d. Stimulating A-delta nerve fibers

46. *If pathology occurs because of a state of "too much" or "not enough," then health would occur because of _____.*

    a. Increased immune activity
    b. Decreased sympathetic arousal response
    c. Effective feedback and adaptive capacity
    d. Tolerance and hardiness

47. *According to Hans Selye the body's response to stress is called the _____.*

    a. Fight-or-flight response
    b. Resistance reaction
    c. Exhaustion phase
    d. General adaptation syndrome

48. *People who perceive an event as a threat activate the alarm reaction. What is the first response?*

    a. The sympathetic centers activate
    b. The hypothalamus is stimulated
    c. The adrenal cortex releases glucocorticoid
    d. The adrenal medulla releases epinephrine

49. *A common breathing disturbance in excessive or long-term stress is _____.*

    a. Hyperventilation syndrome
    b. Immune suppression
    c. Gastritis
    d. Tetany

50. *Many aspects of ancient healing wisdom are being shown as valid stress management strategies due to _____.*

    a. Support of increased heart rate
    b. Reduction in sympathetic arousal
    c. Increase in glucocorticoids
    d. Increase in blood glucose levels

51. *At which life stage are we best able to maintain effective homeostasis?*

    a. Birth to 3 years old
    b. 4 years old to 12 years old
    c. Adolescence to midlife
    d. 65 years old and older

Answers are on pages 14–16.

Answers and Discussion

1. **c**
   Factual recall
   Rationale: Eastern bodywork theory has homeostasis as a primary philosophy. The ability to define the words in the question and the four possible answers is necessary.

2. **d**
   Factual recall
   Rationale: The question is a definition of dosha.

3. **b**
   Factual recall
   Rationale: The question asks for a function of vata.

4. **c**
   Application and concept identification
   Rationale: Information exchange is necessary for a feedback loop, and feedback loops support homeostasis.

5. **c**
   Factual recall
   Rationale: The question is a definition of stress.

6. **d**
   Factual recall
   Rationale: The question lists the parts of a feedback loop.

7. **b**
   Factual recall
   Rationale: The question gives a definition of negative feedback.

8. **d**
   Application and concept identification
   Rationale: The question is asking for a connection between massage and feedback loops. To understand the question the terms need to be defined and an understanding of the physiologic response to massage stimuli is required. Massage and bodywork methods are initially processed as a stress stimulus.

9. **a**
   Application and concept identification
   Rationale: The three incorrect answers misuse the terminology. The correct answer identifies how massage begins a feedback process.

10. **c**
    Factual recall
    Rationale: Definition of the terms in the question and answers is necessary to analyze for the correct answer. Negative feedback keeps body rhythms organized.

11. **d**
    Application and concept identification
    Rationale: Three concepts are correlated—biologic rhythms, entrainment, and autonomic nervous system functions. All three must be connected correctly. Only answer d is correct.

12. **b**
    Application and concept identification
    Rationale: The question asks for justification of physiologic outcome of massage. The terms need to be defined correctly to answer the question. Two processes take place to provide the outcome described in the question, and only answer b identifies both.

13. **b**
    Application and concept identification
    Rationale: Four concepts are described in the question and correct answer. All four must be correlated correctly: relaxation, breathing, entrainment, and respiration as a biologic oscillator. Only answer b connects the concepts correctly.

14. **c**
    Factual recall
    Rationale: The Eastern thought justifying bodywork modalities very often corresponds with anatomy and physiology described in Western science. This question described this type of relationship.

15. **a**
    Factual recall
    Rationale: The question gives a definition of health.

16. **b**
    Factual recall
    Rationale: The question gives a definition of pathology. All the terms need to be defined to correctly answer the question and identify wrong answers.

17. **d**
    Factual recall
    Rationale: The question gives a definition of a syndrome. All the terms need to be defined to correctly answer the question and identify wrong answers.

18. **c**
Factual recall
Rationale: The question gives a definition of chronic. All the terms need to be defined to correctly answer the question and identify wrong answers.

19. **b**
Factual recall
Rationale: Malnutrition is the only possible answer that would describe disease susceptibility. All the terms need to be defined to correctly answer the question and identify wrong answers.

20. **a**
Factual recall
Rationale: Parasites is the only answer that fits the criteria of being a pathogenic organism.

21. **c**
Factual recall
Rationale: All the terms need to be defined to correctly answer the question and identify wrong answers. A neoplasm is abnormal tissue growth, hyperplasia is an uncontrolled increase in cell number, and the definition of benign includes growths that are contained and encapsulated as opposed to malignant, which is a nonencapsulated mass.

22. **d**
Factual recall
Rationale: The question gives a definition of anaplasia. All the terms need to be defined to correctly answer the question and identify wrong answers.

23. **d**
Factual recall
Rationale: The question gives a definition of inflammation. All the terms need to be defined to correctly answer the question and identify wrong answers.

24. **b**
Factual recall
Rationale: The question asks for the function of exudates, which is to dilute irritants causing inflammation.

25. **a**
Factual recall
Rationale: Histamine is a vasodilator. All the terms need to be defined to correctly answer the question and identify wrong answers.

26. **b**
Factual recall
Rationale: The correct answer describes the function of increased fluid volume during inflammation. All the terms need to be defined to correctly answer the question and identify wrong answers.

27. **c**
Factual recall
Rationale: The terms need to be defined correctly to answer the question. When this is done, the only correct answer is answer c.

28. **b**
Factual recall
Rationale: The terms need to be defined correctly to answer the question. Tissue repair resulting in a scar is replacement.

29. **d**
Factual recall
Rationale: The terms need to be defined correctly to answer the question indicating that collagen is the major component of scar tissue.

30. **c**
Application and concept identification
Rationale: The question asks for the physiologic outcome of certain massage methods to resolve a type of chronic inflammation. This is done by creating a controlled therapeutic inflammation, and friction, stretching, and pulling tissue are the best methods to accomplish this.

31. **c**
Application and concept identification
Rationale: The conditions described in the question represent contraindications to the use of therapeutic inflammation since the body is unable to resolve inflammatory processes.

32. **b**
Factual recall
Rationale: The correct answer describes risk factors appropriately while the incorrect answers are not correlated to the information in the question.

33. **d**
Factual recall
Rationale: Pain is the chief complaint over the other three listed.

34. **a**
Factual recall
Rationale: The question describes a function of pain.

35. **c**
Factual recall
Rationale: Nociceptors are the sensory mechanisms for pain perception. The other terms are incorrect.

36. **d**
Factual recall
Rationale: The question is the definition of deep pain.

37. **c**
Factual recall
Rationale: Organ pain is perceived as an aching. It is important to differentiate the types of pain so that appropriate referral can be made to the physician.

38. **c**
Factual recall
Rationale: The soma relates to the soft tissue elements described in the question.

39. **a**
Factual recall
Rationale: The question is a definition of counterirritation.

40. **d**
Factual recall
Rationale: The question is a definition of referred pain.

41. **d**
Clinical reasoning/synthesis
Rationale: To answer this question use factual information of referred pain patterns to make a decision about what the information might mean. The facts of the question describe the referred pain pattern of the gallbladder.

42. **b**
Application and concept identification
Rationale: The question asks for a correlation between symptoms and referred pain patterns. The kidney most often refers pain to the lumbar area.

43. **c**
Clinical reasoning/synthesis
Rationale: The question is asking for an explanation for a client behavior, in this instance high pain tolerance. The other answers describe either a massage outcome or a response that is contradictory (i.e., if endorphin levels drop, then the client would be more aware of pain, not less aware of pain).

44. **a**
Application and concept identification
Rationale: The terms must be understood to answer the question. The only answer that makes sense in relationship to the question is answer a.

45. **c**
Factual recall
Rationale: Effect of aspirin on pain perception is through effects on prostaglandin.

46. **c**
Application and concept identification
Rationale: The question uses a comparison or contrast structure to define health as the ability to use feedback mechanisms allowing the body to adapt to stress and restore itself.

47. **d**
Factual recall
Rationale: The question is a definition of the general adaptation syndrome.

48. **b**
Application and concept identification
Rationale: The hypothalamus is the first responder to the perception of threat, and then the hypothalamus releases corticotrophin-releasing hormones.

49. **a**
Factual recall
Rationale: The only term listed in the answer that relates to breathing is hyperventilation syndrome, which is a common functional disturbance of the stress response.

50. **b**
Application and concept identification
Rationale: All of the answers except b indicate an increase in the stress response instead of a method to manage stress.

51. **c**
Factual recall
Rationale: The very young and the old are not as able to maintain homeostasis, while young adults and those in the middle of life are the most able to stay healthy.

3

Medical Terminology

Questions

1. *A prefix, root, or suffix is based on Latin or Greek* _____.

   a. Grammar
   b. Basic word meaning
   c. Word elements
   d. Sentence structure

2. *The prefix auto- means* _____.

   a. Self
   b. Hear
   c. Against
   d. Both sides

3. *The prefix meaning against or opposite is* _____.

   a. Circum-
   b. Caud-
   c. Contra-
   d. Brach-

4. *The prefix mal- means* _____.

   a. Large
   b. One or single
   c. Form or shape
   d. Illness or disease

5. *The prefix for hard is* _____.

   a. Schist(o)-
   b. Sepsi-
   c. Scler(o)-
   d. Kyph(o)-

6. *The root word pneum(o)- means* _____.

   a. Vein
   b. Lung or gas
   c. Chest
   d. Breathing

7. *The root word for kidney is* _____.

   a. Nephr(o)-
   b. Neur(o)-
   c. Uro-
   d. Phleb(o)-

8. *The suffix for pain is* _____.

   a. -asis
   b. -ase
   c. -algia
   d. -emia

9. *The suffix -pnea means* _____.

   a. To breathe
   b. Paralysis
   c. Putrefaction
   d. Little

10. *The use of abbreviations in charting* _____.

    a. Is universally understood
    b. Is more time consuming
    c. Requires a deciphering key
    d. Clearly communicates information

Answers are on pages 20–21.

11. The ability to think through and justify an intervention process is called _____.

    a. History taking
    b. Assessment
    c. Database collection
    d. Clinical reasoning

12. The history-taking interview provides data for which part of the SOAP note charting process?

    a. Subjective data
    b. Objective data
    c. Analysis
    d. Plan

13. The aspect of the physical assessment that identifies altered movement patterns is _____.

    a. Visual assessment
    b. Functional assessment
    c. Palpation assessment
    d. Objective assessment

14. Physical assessment provides data for which SOAP charting area?

    a. Subjective data
    b. Objective data
    c. Analysis
    d. Plan

15. In order for the data collected during the interview process and physical assessment to be focused to a particular outcome for the client, the information must be _____.

    a. Recorded in a SOAP note
    b. Communicated to the client
    c. Analyzed using a logical process
    d. Written in medical terminology

16. Potential referral to another health care professional is based on which part of the clinical reasoning process?

    a. Assessment of data
    b. Data collection
    c. Plan development
    d. History interview

17. The head, neck, trunk, and spinal cord are considered to be _____.

    a. Appendicular
    b. Thoracic
    c. Axial
    d. Ventral

18. The bladder is located in which region of the abdomen?

    a. Epigastric
    b. Umbilical
    c. Left iliac
    d. Hypogastric

19. The liver is located in which quadrant?

    a. Right upper
    b. Left upper
    c. Right lower
    d. Left lower

20. Which movement decreases the angle of a joint?

    a. Flexion
    b. Extension
    c. Retraction
    d. Adduction

21. The term meaning on the same side is _____.

    a. Lateral
    b. Contralateral
    c. Ipsilateral
    d. Dextral

22. The term meaning closer to the trunk or point of origin is _____.

    a. Anterior
    b. Posterior
    c. Distal
    d. Proximal

23. *Many ancient healing practices were developed based on _____.*

    a. Measurement of concrete functions
    b. Experiential observation
    c. Scientific methods
    d. Meridian system

24. *A commonality of the point phenomena is _____.*

    a. All points are located over motor points
    b. All refer pain patterns
    c. They are located over A-delta and C afferent nerve fibers
    d. They are located in meridian pathways

25. *The cutaneous/visceral reflexes are correlated with which Chinese medicine concept?*

    a. Essential substances
    b. Pernicious influences
    c. Organ systems
    d. Five elements

Answers are on pages 20–21.

Answers and Discussion

1. **c**
   Factual recall
   Rationale: The question is a definition.

2. **a**
   Factual recall
   Rationale: The question is a definition and is representative of this type of question. Any of the word elements can appear in a question structure; therefore, all would need to be understood.

3. **c**
   Factual recall
   Rationale: The question is a definition and is representative of this type of question. Any of the word elements can appear in a question structure; therefore, all would need to be understood.

4. **d**
   Factual recall
   Rationale: The question is a definition and is representative of this type of question. Any of the word elements can appear in a question structure; therefore, all would need to be understood.

5. **c**
   Factual recall
   Rationale: The question is a definition and is representative of this type of question. Any of the word elements can appear in a question structure; therefore, all would need to be understood.

6. **b**
   Factual recall
   Rationale: The question is a definition and is representative of this type of question. Any of the word elements can appear in a question structure; therefore, all would need to be understood.

7. **a**
   Factual recall
   Rationale: The question is a definition and is representative of this type of question. Any of the word elements can appear in a question structure; therefore, all would need to be understood.

8. **c**
   Factual recall
   Rationale: The question is a definition and is representative of this type of question. Any of the word elements can appear in a question structure; therefore, all would need to be understood.

9. **a**
   Factual recall
   Rationale: The question is a definition and is representative of this type of question. Any of the word elements can appear in a question structure; therefore, all would need to be understood.

10. **c**
    Application and concept identification
    Rationale: Whenever nonstandard abbreviations are used, a deciphering key is necessary.

11. **d**
    Factual recall
    Rationale: The question is a definition of clinical reasoning.

12. **a**
    Factual recall
    Rationale: The question is a definition of subjective data.

13. **b**
    Factual recall
    Rationale: The question is a definition of functional assessment. As in all questions, it is important to define all terms to properly analyze information for the correct answer.

14. **b**
    Factual recall
    Rationale: The question is a definition of objective data.

15. **c**
    Factual recall
    Rationale: The question is a definition of analysis.

16. **c**
    Factual recall
    Rationale: The question is representative of information in a plan.

17. **c**
    Factual recall
    Rationale: The question is a list of structures in the axial area.

18. **d**
    Factual recall
    Rationale: The question is representative of information about the structural plan of the body.

19. **a**
    Factual recall
    Rationale: The question is representative of information about the structural plan of the body.

20. **a**
Factual recall
Rationale: The question is representative of information about the movement of the body.

21. **c**
Factual recall
Rationale: The question is representative of information about the directional terms.

22. **d**
Factual recall
Rationale: The question is representative of information about the directional terms.

23. **b**
Application and concept identification
Rationale: Accumulated experience provided the base for consistent patterns observed by ancient healers.

24. **c**
Factual recall
Rationale: The question is representative of information that correlates Eastern theory with Western science. Many different systems evolved a point theory, and the location of these points consistently falls over nerves and sensory receptors.

25. **c**
Application and concept identification
Rationale: The three incorrect answers describe Chinese concepts that are not related to the cutaneous/visceral reflexes. Only answer c is logical if the definitions of essential substances, pernicious influences, and five elements theory are understood. This question is representative of usage of Eastern terminology.

4

Nervous System Basics and Central Nervous System

Questions

1. Which of the following is a principle of quantum physics?

   a. Predicts events
   b. Can be pictured
   c. Describes statistical behavior of systems and groups
   d. Holds that we can observe something without changing it

2. The nervous system and the endocrine system reflect quantum properties because _____.

   a. Predictable physiologic outcomes are constant
   b. Feedback loops reliably affect outcomes
   c. Linear pathways of affect are constant
   d. Tendency for response is most accurate

3. A function of neuroglia is to _____.

   a. Transmit signals to the cell body
   b. Carry signals away from the cell body
   c. Conduct signals from one neuron to another
   d. Support and protect neurons

4. Neurilemma is formed by _____.

   a. Schwann cells
   b. Myelin
   c. Dendrites
   d. Axons

5. Neurons that conduct signals to the central nervous system are _____.

   a. Sensory neurons
   b. Motor neurons
   c. Interneurons
   d. Nodes of Ranvier

6. Sensory stimulation of massage causes a chemical change in a neuron called _____.

   a. Action potential
   b. Refractory period
   c. Depolarization
   d. Saltatory conduction

7. When a neuron is positively charged on the outside of the cell membrane and negatively charged on the inside, it has _____.

   a. Saltatory conduction
   b. Membrane potential
   c. Action potential
   d. Refractory potential

8. *Which phase of nerve signal conduction is related to muscle energy methods of massage that use some sort of muscle contraction to prepare the muscle to relax and lengthen?*

   a. Action potential
   b. Refractory period
   c. Depolarization
   d. Saltatory conduction

9. *Nerve axon repair in the peripheral nervous system is produced by _____.*

   a. Oligodendrocytes
   b. Synaptic vesicles
   c. Neurilemma
   d. Endoplasmic reticulum

10. *Action potential between neurons occurs across the synaptic cleft because of _____.*

   a. Neurotransmitters
   b. Postsynaptic membrane
   c. Anterograde transport
   d. Nodes of Ranvier

11. *The neurotransmitter that primarily excites the skeletal muscles is _____.*

   a. Dopamine
   b. Acetylcholine
   c. Cholecystokinin
   d. Somatostatin

12. *A person is clumsy and has a dull or foggy mind in terms of understanding information and making decisions. Which of the following neurotransmitters may be involved?*

   a. Norepinephrine
   b. Histamine
   c. Glutamate
   d. Dopamine

13. *Neurotransmitters work in excitatory and inhibitory pairs. Which of the following would provide a balancing action for enkephalin?*

   a. Somatostatin
   b. Substance P
   c. Serotonin
   d. GABA

14. *A massage client reports that after the massage she had some itchy areas of skin. Her clothes felt rough against her skin. Which neurotransmitter may be involved?*

   a. Histamine
   b. Acetylcholine
   c. Epinephrine
   d. CCK

15. *A client reports before the massage that his mind is agitated. He feels like he wants to scream. He is talking loudly and pacing. After the massage he feels calmer and wants a nap. Which neurotransmitter is largely responsible for the mood change?*

   a. Norepinephrine
   b. Dopamine
   c. Serotonin
   d. Substance P

16. *The purpose of therapeutic (feel good) pain during massage to manage undesirable pain is to stimulate which neurotransmitters?*

   a. Serotonin and endorphin
   b. Epinephrine and histamine
   c. Acetylcholine and dopamine
   d. Histamine and substance P

17. *The portion of the brain that interprets sensory data and compares it against past memories and experiences is the _____.*

   a. Ventricles
   b. Pineal body
   c. Cerebrum
   d. Temporal lobe

18. The structure that connects the right and left hemispheres of the cerebrum is the _____.

    a. Basal ganglia
    b. Sulcus
    c. Corpus callosum
    d. Longitudinal fissure

19. The primary area of the brain that would process the pain/pleasure aspect of massage is the _____.

    a. Frontal lobe
    b. Parietal lobe
    c. Temporal lobe
    d. Occipital lobe

20. Activities that occur in the cerebrum after sensory signals are received and before motor responses are sent are called _____.

    a. Integrative functions
    b. Convolutions
    c. Inhibitory functions
    d. Activating systems

21. Conscious awareness of our environment is related to what structural and functional area of the brain?

    a. Primary motor cortex
    b. Reticular activating system
    c. Sensory associate cortex
    d. Temporal pole

22. The area of the brain responsible for motor sequencing, posture in relationship to the environment, and processing spatial relations is the _____.

    a. Limbic lobes
    b. Temporal lobes
    c. Frontal lobes
    d. Parietal lobes

23. States of higher consciousness are related to _____.

    a. Alertness with relaxation
    b. Decreased health states
    c. Increased sympathetic arousal
    d. Depression with pain

24. Uncontrolled emotional display may indicate problems with what brain area?

    a. Basal ganglia
    b. Left hemisphere of the cerebrum
    c. Limbic system
    d. Primary motor area

25. Why do the primary motor and the primary somesthetic sensory areas of the brain interfere with the ability to successfully self-massage areas of the back and limbs?

    a. The largest sensory and motor awareness is in these areas
    b. The distribution of sensory and motor function to the hands is too small to stimulate sensation
    c. The distribution of sensory and motor function is larger to the hands than to the back and limbs
    d. The back and limbs have a predominance of sensory distribution over the motor distribution of the hands

26. Protein synthesis and physical brain changes in the temporal lobes support long-term memory with _____.

    a. State-dependent memory
    b. Engrams
    c. Pleasure states
    d. Entrainment

27. Which of the following drugs is a central nervous system depressant?

    a. Cocaine
    b. Caffeine
    c. Alcohol
    d. Amphetamines

28. Which brain area functions to regulate vital life functions such as heart rate, blood pressure, and breathing?

    a. Midbrain
    b. Pons
    c. Cerebellum
    d. Medulla oblongata

Answers are on pages 27–29.

29. Pleasure states experienced during massage that support mind-body health are processed in what area of the diencephalon?

    a. Thalamus
    b. Pineal body
    c. Meninges
    d. Midbrain

    False brain where the thalamus lies

30. A massage session that incorporates rocking affects the <u>vestibular system</u> including <u>labyrinthine</u> righting reflexes. Which brain area is also stimulated to coordinate appropriate posture?

    a. Cerebellum
    b. Pons
    c. Motor descending tracts
    d. Sensory ascending tracts

31. The protective membrane that adheres to the brain is the _____.

    a. Dura mater
    b. Arachnoid mater
    c. Epidural mater
    d. Pia mater

32. Massage sensations travel on which spinal cord tracts?

    a. Sensory ascending tracts
    b. Motor descending tracts
    c. Corticospinal tracts
    d. Lateral reticulospinal tracts

33. In which pathologic process would massage be most beneficial in assisting in the movement of body fluids?

    a. Upper motor neuron injury
    b. Lower motor neuron injury
    c. Aneurysm
    d. Chorea

34. Research indicates that massage increases the body's availability of the following neurotransmitters—norepinephrine, serotonin, and dopamine. Which central nervous system disorder would be most benefited by massage?

    a. Stroke
    b. Cerebral palsy
    c. Depression
    d. Schizophrenia

#30 Cerebellum maintains proper posture & balance

Answers and Discussion

1. **c**
Factual recall
Rationale: The question is a definition of quantum physics.

2. **d**
Application and concept identification
Rationale: The physiology of these two systems of control is best described in view of quantum mechanics.

3. **d**
Factual recall
Rationale: The correct answer is a primary function of this specialized connective tissue. The three wrong answers describe other nervous system function.

4. **a**
Factual recall
Rationale: Myelin, dendrites, and axons do not form or secrete any substance. Only Schwann cells form myelin and its outer covering called the neurilemma.

5. **a**
Factual recall
Rationale: The question is a definition of sensory neurons. To answer this question the definitions of all of the terms are necessary.

6. **c**
Application and concept identification
Rationale: To answer the question there needs to be an understanding of how nerve conduction functions. Some of these functions are listed in the possible answers. The question asks how massage causes the neuron to transmit a signal. A stimulus such as the pressure of massage causes a change in the charge of one segment of a neuron. This is depolarization.

7. **b**
Factual recall
Rationale: The question is the definition of membrane potential when the nerve is at rest.

8. **b**
Application and concept identification
Rationale: The question is asking for a connection to the application of a bodywork method—muscle energy when a muscle uses contraction to initiate relaxation. The refractory period occurs after a nerve transmission. During this time the nerve does not readily respond to stimuli, allowing the muscle it controls to be lengthened.

9. **c**
Factual recall
Rationale: The question describes a function of neurilemma. It is necessary to define all the terms in the question and answers to correctly answer the question.

10. **a**
Factual recall
Rationale: The question describes a function of neurotransmitters. It is necessary to define all the terms in the question and answers to correctly answer the question.

11. **b**
Factual recall
Rationale: The question describes a function of acetylcholine. It is necessary to define all the terms in the question and answers to correctly answer the question.

12. **d**
Application and concept identification
Rationale: The question describes a function of dopamine in relationship to behavior. It is necessary to define all the terms in the question and answers to correctly answer the question.

13. **b**
Application and concept identification
Rationale: The question provides half of a balancing pair of neurotransmitters. It is necessary to define all the terms in the question and answers to correctly answer the question. Enkephalin inhibits pain signals, and substance P transmits pain signals.

14. **a**
Application and concept identification
Rationale: The question describes a function of histamine in relationship to behavior. It is necessary to define all the terms in the question and answers to correctly answer the question.

15. **c**
Application and concept identification
Rationale: The question describes a function of serotonin in relationship to behavior and in response to massage. It is necessary to define all the terms in the question and answers to correctly answer the question.

16. **a**
    Application and concept identification
    Rationale: The question describes a function of serotonin and endorphin in relationship to massage applications. It is necessary to define all the terms in the question and answers to correctly answer the question.

17. **c**
    Factual recall
    Rationale: The question describes a function of the cerebrum. It is necessary to define all the terms in the question and answers to correctly answer the question.

18. **c**
    Factual recall
    Rationale: The question describes the location of the corpus callosum. It is necessary to define all the terms in the question and answers to correctly answer the question.

19. **b**
    Factual recall
    Rationale: The question describes a function of the parietal lobe. It is necessary to define all the terms in the question and answers to correctly answer the question.

20. **a**
    Factual recall
    Rationale: The question describes integrative functions of the cortex. It is necessary to define all the terms in the question and answers and to know the function of the cerebrum to correctly answer the question.

21. **b**
    Factual recall
    Rationale: The question describes a function of the reticular activating system. It is necessary to define all the terms in the question and answers to correctly answer the question.

22. **d**
    Factual recall
    Rationale: The question describes a function of parietal lobes in the brain. It is necessary to define all the terms in the question and answers to correctly answer the question.

23. **a**
    Application and concept identification
    Rationale: The question asks for an application of central nervous system functions. Only the correct answer is reasonable in relation to the concept of higher consciousness.

24. **c**
    Factual recall
    Rationale: The question describes a function of the limbic system. It is necessary to define all the terms in the question and answers to correctly answer the question.

25. **c**
    Application and concept identification
    Rationale: The question asks for an application of central nervous system function and an interpretation of sensory perception based on sensory and motor distribution in these areas of the brain. Only the correct answer explains the reason for self-massage being less than successful.

26. **b**
    Factual recall
    Rationale: The question describes creation of long-term memory. It is necessary to define all the terms in the question and answers to correctly answer the question.

27. **c**
    Factual recall
    Rationale: The question describes substances that affect the central nervous system. It is necessary to define all the terms in the question and answers to correctly answer the question.

28. **d**
    Factual recall
    Rationale: The question describes a function of the medulla oblongata. It is necessary to define all the terms in the question and answers to correctly answer the question.

29. **a**
    Factual recall
    Rationale: The question describes a function of the thalamus. It is necessary to define all the terms in the question and answers to correctly answer the question.

30. **a**
    Factual recall
    Rationale: The question describes a function of the cerebellum. It is necessary to define all the terms in the question and answers to correctly answer the question.

31. **d**
    Factual recall
    Rationale: The question describes the location of the pia mater. It is necessary to define all the terms in the question and answers to correctly answer the question. The epidural mater is an incorrect use of terms and does not exist.

32. **a**

    Application and concept identification
    Rationale: The question is asking for an under-
    standing of how sensory signals of massage are
    processed. It is necessary to define all the terms
    in the question and answers to correctly answer
    the question.

33. **b**

    Application and concept identification
    Rationale: The question is asking for an under-
    standing of how massage may be indicated for
    pathology of the central nervous system. It is
    necessary to define all the terms in the question
    and answers to correctly answer the question.
    Once the disease processes are understood, then
    the decision needs to be made about which one
    would require assistance in moving fluids in the
    body. Lower motor neuron injury results in
    flaccid muscles, and the pumping action of
    muscles to assist fluid movement is lost.

34. **c**

    Application and concept identification
    Rationale: The question is asking for an under-
    standing of how massage may be indicated for
    pathology of the central nervous system. It is
    necessary to define all the terms in the question
    and answers to correctly answer the question.
    Once the disease processes are understood, then
    the decision needs to be made about which one
    would respond best to a change in neurotrans-
    mitters. Depression may respond to an increase
    in the availability of the neurotransmitters
    described in the question. Schizophrenia may
    temporarily worsen. The other two are not
    directly linked to neurotransmitters.

CHAPTER

5

Peripheral Nervous System

Questions

1. Peripheral nerves that innervate the muscles and skin are known as _____.

   a. Visceral
   b. Afferent
   c. Somatic
   d. Thermal

2. A bundle of axons and dendrites that carry either sensory or motor signals is called a _____.

   a. Neuron
   b. Nerve
   c. Dermatome
   d. Plexus

3. The connective tissue covering that surrounds the fasciculus is called _____.

   a. Endoneurium
   b. Epineurium
   c. Perineurium
   d. Meninges

4. What cranial nerve affects visceral function?

   a. Vagus nerve
   b. Hypoglossal
   c. Trigeminal
   d. Trochlear

5. The dorsal root ganglion contains cell bodies of _____.

   a. Sensory neurons
   b. Motor neurons
   c. Mixed nerves
   d. Cranial nerves

6. The phrenic nerve is part of which plexus?

   a. Cervical
   b. Brachial
   c. Lumbar
   d. Sacral

7. If a client complains of pain in the buttocks and into the lateral side of the leg, which plexus is a potential site of nerve impingement?

   a. Cervical
   b. Brachial
   c. Lumbar
   d. Sacral

8. Pain, tingling, and numbness in the arm and hand may be the result from nerve damage in which plexus?

   a. Cervical
   b. Brachial
   c. Lumbar
   d. Sacral

9. The obturator nerve is found in which plexus?

    a. Cervical
    b. Brachial
    c. Lumbar
    d. Sacral

10. During massage, pain that is not related to specific symptoms radiates around the ear. This indicates excessive pressure on which nerve?

    a. Greater auricular
    b. Thoracodorsal
    c. Medial cutaneous
    d. Pudendal

11. A client complains of pain in the region of the low back and buttocks. Which dermatome nerve distribution might indicate where the nerve impingement is located?

    a. C-7
    b. T-2
    c. C-6
    d. L-2

12. During the history interview a client reports that she almost fell down stairs but caught herself and was able to regain her balance. What type of reflex action was required to accomplish this?

    a. Monosynaptic
    b. Polysynaptic
    c. Patellar
    d. Pacinian

13. Changes in blood pressure are monitored by _____.

    a. Exteroceptors
    b. Proprioceptors
    c. Visceroceptors
    d. Nociceptors

14. Reflexes are most often processed in which part of the CNS?

    a. Cerebrum
    b. Ventricles
    c. Dura
    d. Spinal cord

15. A client is complaining of difficulty hitting a golf ball and describes a sense of timing being off. This could be a result of a disruption in what type of reflex?

    a. Conditioned reflex
    b. Tendon reflex
    c. Stretch reflex
    d. Mono reflex

16. A client is having difficulty being comfortable with the touch of draping material during the massage. He says that he cannot get used to the scratchy feeling. The client may be displaying a reduced ability of sensory receptors to _____.

    a. Send impulses
    b. Adapt to sensation
    c. Remain monosynaptic
    d. Initiate reciprocal inhibition

17. The sensory receptors most affected by deep compression and slow gliding strokes are _____.

    a. Pacinian corpuscles
    b. Root hair plexuses
    c. Merkel's disks
    d. Ruffini's end organs

18. Which of the following receptors is most likely to adapt and cease responding to the sustained compression during massage on one specific area of the body?

    a. Meissner's corpuscles
    b. Thermal receptors
    c. Type II cutaneous mechanoreceptors
    d. Nociceptors

19. Mechanical receptors that provide us with information about position and movement are _____.

    a. Reciprocal inhibition
    b. Thermal receptors
    c. Proprioceptors
    d. Externoreceptors

20. A compressive massage method is applied to the belly of a muscle with the intent of reducing a muscle spasm brought on by a cramp. The receptors most affected are _____.

    a. Joint kinesthetic
    b. Golgi tendon organ
    c. Muscle spindles
    d. Meissner's corpuscles

21. As slow deep effleurage is applied to the left upper thigh, the practitioner notices and the client describes a twitching of the muscles in the back of the opposite leg. What type of reflex has been stimulated?

    a. Stretch reflex
    b. Tendon reflex
    c. Ipsilateral reflex
    d. Contralateral reflex

22. The portion of the autonomic nervous system that supports energy conservation is _____.

    a. Parasympathetic
    b. Peripheral
    c. Somatic
    d. Sympathetic

23. The thoracolumbar division of the autonomic nervous system contains ganglia located _____.

    a. Near the spine
    b. At the effector organs
    c. In the spinal column
    d. In the cranial and sacral areas

24. A client reports being prone to headaches from being in bright light. Bright light has only been a problem in the last few weeks. The client also reports an increase in workload. What might be the function of the ANS that could be responsible for the sensitivity to light?

    a. Parasympathetic dilation of the pupil
    b. Sympathetic dilation of the pupil
    c. Parasympathetic contraction of the pupil
    d. Sympathetic contraction of the pupil

25. A client requests an outcome from the massage session that includes a good night's sleep and less fidgeting. The massage session would then need to be designed to accomplish what?

    a. Cranial sacral plexus inhibition
    b. Parasympathetic inhibition
    c. Sympathetic inhibition
    d. Sympathetic dominance

26. The release of epinephrine into the system is called _____.

    a. Parasympathetic dominance
    b. Adrenergic stimulation
    c. Sympathetic inhibition
    d. Parasympathetic facilitation

27. The primary neurotransmitter of the parasympathetic system is _____.

    a. Acetylcholine
    b. Epinephrine
    c. Norepinephrine
    d. Adrenaline

28. The sympathetic chain ganglia are located in an area similar to the Back-shu points on which meridian?

    a. Spleen
    b. Kidney
    c. Liver
    d. Bladder

29. Acupuncture points are often located in the same area as _____.

    a. Motor points
    b. Synapse
    c. Root hair plexus
    d. Myotomes

30. Research seems to indicate that one of the most noticeable beneficial effects of acupuncture is that it produces what physiologic response?

    a. Parasympathetic inhibition
    b. Sympathetic inhibition
    c. Inhibition of endorphins
    d. Sympathetic facilitation

Answers are on pages 36–39.

31. Which of the following physiologic effects do massage and acupuncture share?

   a. Increases sympathetic arousal
   b. Decreases levels of endorphins
   c. Blocks release of substance P
   d. Decreases parasympathetic arousal

32. A client appears particularly agitated during the initial history interview. What is the best voice pattern to use to calm the client and best ensure that the client understands you?

   a. A slow high pitch
   b. A fast deep pitch
   c. A slow deep pitch
   d. A fast deep pitch

33. The bones in the ear that respond to vibration of the tympanic membrane are called _____.

   a. Pinna
   b. Ossicles
   c. Cochlea
   d. Corti

34. The massage method that most affects the inner ear balance mechanisms is _____.

   a. Tapotement
   b. Compression
   c. Friction
   d. Rocking

35. When vision records a change in the environment, it causes a signal to be sent to which part of the brain?

   a. Frontal lobe
   b. Cerebellum
   c. Ventricles
   d. Sulcus

36. Righting reflexes combine information from vision and the vestibular mechanisms to maintain _____.

   a. Baroreceptors
   b. Equilibrium
   c. Sclera
   d. Vertigo

37. A client indicates in the history interview that he is prone to motion sickness. Which massage methods should be avoided?

   a. Active joint movement
   b. Stretching
   c. Rocking
   d. Compression

38. Which of the following senses exerts the strongest influence on the emotional limbic system?

   a. Smell
   b. Taste
   c. Hearing
   d. Sight

39. Which of the following is a structure of the nose?

   a. Ciliary body
   b. Canthus
   c. Turbinate
   d. Sclera

40. A client complains of radiating pain down the arm into the elbow and fingers. The client has not been evaluated by a physician, so a referral is indicated. Which diagnosis by the physician would be most helped by massage?

   a. Guillain-Barré syndrome
   b. Brachial plexus entrapment
   c. Cervical plexus compression
   d. Osteoporosis

41. A client reports having herpes zoster and is experiencing pain. Which of the following would be the best massage approach?

   a. A full-body 1-hour massage with attention to universal precautions that uses tapotement, active joint movement, and fractioning methods
   b. A full-body massage lasting 1½ hours that avoids the area of the rash and that actively engages the client in muscle energy lengthening and stretching
   c. A seated massage that lasts for 15 minutes
   d. A full-body, 1-hour massage that avoids the area of the rash with attention to universal precautions and a focus toward relaxation

42. *A client seeks massage after a diagnosis of neuralgia in the left leg. Which of the following would be a realistic therapeutic massage outcome?*

    a. Reduction of pain and regeneration
    b. Long-term symptom decrease
    c. Short-term pain management
    d. Short-term regeneration

43. *A client is complaining of a recent inability to sleep and a feeling of agitation and reports concern over a change in management systems at work. The physician diagnosis was exogenous anxiety. Which of the following treatment plans is most appropriate?*

    a. Mild exercise program, therapeutic massage, and a medication such as imipramine to control symptoms
    b. A hypoventilation syndrome management program including massage and chiropractic manipulation
    c. A mild exercise program, cognitive behavioral therapy, short-term use of diazepam, and relaxation massage
    d. Therapeutic massage, meditation, increase in caffeine consumption, and bed rest

Answers are on pages 36–39.

Answers and Discussion

1. **c**
   Factual recall
   Rationale: The question is a definition of somatic nerves.

2. **b**
   Factual recall
   Rationale: The question is a definition of nerves.

3. **a**
   Factual recall
   Rationale: The question uses terminology that would have to be defined to identify the correct answer.

4. **a**
   Factual recall
   Rationale: The question is representative of cranial nerve function. All of the functions of cranial nerves would be needed to correctly answer the question.

5. **a**
   Factual recall
   Rationale: The question is representative of peripheral nervous system anatomy. A strong knowledge of the terminology and function of this anatomy would be needed to correctly answer the question.

6. **a**
   Factual recall
   Rationale: The question is representative of peripheral nervous system anatomy. A strong knowledge of the terminology and function of this anatomy would be needed to correctly answer the question.

7. **c**
   Application and concept identification
   Rationale: Answering this question depends on an understanding of peripheral nervous system anatomy. Symptoms indicate that the lumbar plexus is involved.

8. **b**
   Application and concept identification
   Rationale: Answering this question depends on an understanding of peripheral nervous system anatomy. Symptoms indicate that the brachial plexus is involved.

9. **c**
   Factual recall
   Rationale: The question is representative of peripheral nervous system anatomy.

10. **a**
    Application and concept identification
    Rationale: Answering this question depends on an understanding of peripheral nervous system anatomy. Symptoms described in the question are from inappropriate pressure on the greater auricular nerve.

11. **d**
    Application and concept identification
    Rationale: Answering this question depends on an understanding of peripheral nervous system anatomy. Symptoms indicate that a range in dermatome distribution between L-1 and L-3 is likely. Answer d is the only answer that represents this area.

12. **b**
    Application and concept identification
    Rationale: Answering this question depends on an understanding of peripheral nervous system reflex functions. Also required is interpretation of the word elements. Mono means one and poly means many. It takes many reflex actions to regain balance.

13. **c**
    Factual recall
    Rationale: The question is representative of peripheral nervous system function. A strong knowledge of the terminology would be needed to correctly answer the question. Blood pressure is monitored by visceroceptors that detect changes in the internal body environment.

14. **d**
    Factual recall
    Rationale: The question is representative of peripheral nervous system anatomy and physiology. A strong knowledge of the terminology and function of this anatomy would be needed to correctly answer the question. Most reflexes do not make their way past the brainstem, so the spinal cord is the correct answer.

15. **a**

Clinical reasoning/synthesis

Rationale: A decision based on factual data is required to correctly answer the question. The facts presented in the question indicate that the person has a learned training effect to golf. Coordination is disrupted, described as timing being off. Knowledge of the types of reflexes is necessary to choose the best answer. Golf is something learned, so the conditioned reflex is the best answer. Mono reflex does not exist. The tendon and stretch reflex are more involved in muscle tone.

16. **b**

Application and concept identification

Rationale: The question describes sensations that indicate that the client is not getting used to the draping material. The nervous system's ability to adapt to sensation is what allows the body to tolerate ongoing sensation.

17. **d**

Application and concept identification

Rationale: The question is asking for a connection between massage methods that create deep compressive forces and the sensory receptor affected. This is important so that correct methods can be used to generate the type of sensation that specific receptors identify and respond to. Ruffini's end organs would respond to compressive force. The other mechanical sensory receptors listed respond more to light touch.

18. **a**

Application and concept identification

Rationale: The question is asking for a connection between massage methods that create deep compressive forces and the sensory receptor affected. This is important so that correct methods can be used to generate the type of sensation that specific receptors identify and respond to. Meissner's corpuscles adapt quickly.

19. **c**

Factual recall

Rationale: The question is representative of peripheral nervous system anatomy and physiology. A strong knowledge of the terminology and function of this anatomy would be needed to correctly answer the question. The question is the definition of a proprioceptor.

20. **c**

Application and concept identification

Rationale: The question is asking for a connection between massage methods that create compressive forces and the sensory receptor affected and location of that receptor. This is important so that correct methods can be used to generate the type of sensation that specific receptors identify and respond to. Muscle spindles are located primarily in the belly of the muscle and are active when a muscle cramps.

21. **d**

Application and concept identification

Rationale: The question is asking for a connection between massage methods and reflex responses. It is necessary to understand all the reflex patterns listed as possible answers. Since the question describes a pattern involving opposite sides of the body, the contralateral reflex is the correct answer.

22. **a**

Factual recall

Rationale: The question is representative of autonomic nervous system anatomy and physiology. A strong knowledge of the terminology and function of this anatomy would be needed to correctly answer the question. The question describes a function of the parasympathetic system.

23. **a**

Factual recall

Rationale: The question is representative of ANS nervous system anatomy and physiology. A strong knowledge of the terminology and function of this anatomy would be needed to correctly answer the question. The question describes the location of sympathetic nerves and ganglia near the spine.

24. **b**

Clinical reasoning/synthesis

Rationale: The question presents a case that asks for a reason for light sensitivity combined with headache. The facts of the question need to be analyzed. They are: headache brought on by bright light, recent onset, and increased job stress. Next the various responses of the ANS have to be identified in relation to the facts. Increased workload is likely to stimulate sympathetic dominance. An effect of this is pupil dilation, which would increase light sensitivity. The incorrect answers do not describe correct function of the ANS.

25. **c**
    Application and concept identification
    Rationale: The question is asking for a connection between massage methods and changes in the ANS. It is necessary to understand all the reflex patterns listed as possible answers. Since the question describes a pattern of parasympathetic dominance, massage would have to be designed to inhibit sympathetic activation.

26. **b**
    Factual recall
    Rationale: The question is representative of ANS nervous system physiology. A strong knowledge of the terminology and function of this physiology would be needed to correctly answer the question. The term adrenergic is used to describe sympathetic stimulation, and epinephrine is one of the neurotransmitters involved.

27. **a**
    Factual recall
    Rationale: The question is representative of ANS nervous system physiology. A strong knowledge of the terminology and function of this physiology would be needed to correctly answer the question. The main neurotransmitter of the parasympathetic system is acetylcholine.

28. **d**
    Application and concept identification
    Rationale: The question is asking for a connection between the anatomy of the ANS and the traditional meridian system.

29. **a**
    Application and concept identification
    Rationale: The question is asking for a connection between the anatomy of the peripheral nervous system and the traditional acupuncture system.

30. **b**
    Application and concept identification
    Rationale: The question is asking for a connection between the physiology of the ANS and the traditional acupuncture system. When acupuncture is used, parasympathetic dominance usually is evident, so inhibition of the sympathetic functions would also be evident.

31. **c**
    Application and concept identification
    Rationale: The question is asking for a connection among massage effects, the physiology of the ANS, and the traditional acupuncture system. Research indicates that both massage and acupuncture inhibit substance P.

32. **c**
    Application and concept identification
    Rationale: The question is asking for a connection between the physiology of hearing and the use of voice tone. High-pitched fast speaking indicates and can create sympathetic arousal. A slow deep pitch is more calming.

33. **b**
    Factual recall
    Rationale: Answering the question requires an understanding of the terminology in the question and possible answers. The terms in the answers are all related to the ear, but only the term ossicles describes the bones.

34. **d**
    Application and concept identification
    Rationale: The question is asking for a connection between the vestibule mechanism and massage application. The rocking of the head in particular affects this system.

35. **a**
    Factual recall
    Rationale: Answering the question requires an understanding of the terminology in the question and possible answers and the function of these areas. The question asks for a specific visual interpretation, which is processed in the frontal lobes.

36. **b**
    Factual recall
    Rationale: Answering the question requires an understanding of the terminology in the question and possible answers and the functions of these areas. The only logical answer is answer b.

37. **c**
    Application and concept identification
    Rationale: The question is asking for a connection between the vestibule mechanism, pathology, and massage application. Rocking of the head in particular can result in motion sickness.

38. **a**
    Factual recall
    Rationale: Answering the question requires an understanding of the terminology in the question and possible answers and the functions of these areas. The only logical answer is answer a.

39. **c**
    Factual recall
    Rationale: The question asks for identification of terminology. Only the turbinate is located in the nose.

40. **b**
    Clinical reasoning/synthesis
    Rationale: The question is asking for identification of symptoms to support a referral. The facts of the question indicate brachial plexus involvement.

41. **d**
    Clinical reasoning/synthesis
    Rationale: The question is representative of a decision based on pathology. The question is asking for identification of symptoms to support an appropriate massage intervention The facts of the question include a current outbreak of herpes zoster and pain. Each of the answers is a possible approach and would have to be analyzed to determine the best answer. The outcome would be increased tolerance to pain and reduced pain perception. These outcomes are best achieved with parasympathetic dominance and an increase in serotonin and endorphins. In addition, appropriate sanitation is a factor. The client is also immune compromised since an active pathology is present. Only answer d addresses all these issues.

42. **c**
    Clinical reasoning/synthesis
    Rationale: The question is asking for the development of realistic outcomes for massage intervention. The possible answers have to be analyzed to identify which one is best in relation to the facts of the question. The only fact is a diagnosis of neuralgia, which would have to be researched. Neuralgia is a noninflammatory disorder of the nerve resulting in pain. Nerve pain is difficult to manage. The only logical answer is answer c.

43. **c**
    Clinical reasoning/synthesis
    Rationale: The question is representative of a decision based on pathology. The question is asking for identification of symptoms to support an appropriate massage intervention. The facts of the question include: recent sleep disturbance, feeling agitated, work stress, and a diagnosis of exogenous anxiety. Information about exogenous anxiety becomes part of the factual information and indicates that the client is reacting to changes in the environment. Each of the treatment plans offered needs to be analyzed to identify which one best addresses the needs of the client. In addition, information about standard treatment protocols including use of medication is necessary. For this type of reactive anxiety, short-term therapy and medication use are usually successful. Massage would need to support these interventions. The only logical treatment plan is given in answer c.

hormone - substance originating in an organ, glad, or body part that is conveyed the the blood to another body that part to incr chemically stimulating

6

Endocrine System

Questions

1. Which of the following ancient healing systems most correlates with the endocrine system?

   a. Meridian system
   b. Five elements
   c. Doshas
   d. Chakra system

2. Which of the following most accurately describes hormones?

   a. Secreted from exocrine glands
   b. Found in the synapse
   c. Transported in the blood
   d. Secretion regulated by positive feedback

3. A client is experiencing lingering anxiety from a minor auto accident 4 hours ago. What difference between the nervous system and the endocrine system would explain this condition?

   a. The nervous system is short acting and the endocrine system is long acting
   b. The endocrine system is short acting and the nervous system is long acting
   c. The nervous system transports hormones more consistently through blood and tissues
   d. Neurotransmitters have a long duration of effect and hormones are short acting

4. A primary action of hormones is _____.

   a. Increasing or decreasing cellular processes
   b. Supporting positive feedback control of homeostasis
   c. Inhibiting synaptic uptake of neurotransmitters
   d. Suppressing tropic effects of cellular processes

5. Hypersecretion refers to _____.

   a. Normal decrease in endocrine secretion
   b. Abnormal decrease in endocrine secretion
   c. Normal increase in endocrine secretion
   d. Abnormal increase in endocrine secretion

6. Which of the following translates nerve impulses into hormone secretions by endocrine glands?

   a. The limbic system
   b. The pituitary gland
   c. The hypothalamus
   d. The adrenal glands

hypothalamus - regulates H₂O body temp, appetite hormone Releasing by the that control or inhibit

7. *An elderly client with a history of slow tissue healing and gradual weight loss begins to stabilize her weight and increase her ability to heal skin abrasions after receiving a weekly massage for 3 months. Which of the following offers the most concrete explanation for this outcome?*

   (a.) Massage influences positive feedback mechanism to decrease adrenal output

   (b.) Massage supports hypothalamic release of growth hormone–releasing hormone

   c. Massage changes sleep patterns to increase dopamine influence

   d. Massage beneficially influences tissue transport systems of neurotransmitters from endocrine tissues

8. *The pituitary gland is a primary source of _____.*

   (a.) Tropic hormones

   b. Melatonin

   c. Adrenergic hormones

   d. Pitocin

9. *Which of the following supports growth hormone function in the adult?*

   a. High blood sugar

   (b) Loving relationships

   c. Disrupted sleep

   d. Lack of exercise

10. *Which of the following anterior pituitary hormones can be positively influenced by cold hydrotherapy applications?*

    a. Melanocyte-stimulating hormone

    b. Follicle-stimulating hormone

    (c) Thyroid-stimulating hormone

    d. Luteinizing hormone

11. *A 38-year-old female client describes symptoms of constipation, increased edema, sensitivity to cold, muscle and joint pain, and hair loss. She indicates that there is an increase in stress in her life; she is tired and seems unable to cope as effectively as before. She had a general physical examination within the last 6 months but no specific tests were done. Based on these symptoms, which condition might suggest a need for referral?*

    a. Exophthalmos → *abnormal protrusion of eyeball*

    (b.) Hypothyroidism

    c. Hyperthyroidism

    d. Hypocalcemic tetany *abnormal blood calcium Sym → renal failure*

    [margin note: *graves disease*]

12. *A type 2 diabetic wishes to become a client for therapeutic massage. The physician is supportive. Which of the following statements is most accurate as a basic understanding of type 2 diabetes?*

    a. There is a disruption of insulin production from the islet cells of the pituitary gland

    b. Insulin is a powerful diuretic, so increased edema is a warning sign of diabetic coma

    (c.) Insulin is released when levels of blood sugar, amino acids, and fatty acids rise

    d. Glucagon facilitates the ability of insulin to transport glucose across the cell membrane

13. *Which of the following hormones extends the response of the fight or flight produced by the sympathetic autonomic nervous system?*

    (a.) Epinephrine *actured by SAN - maintain blood pressure - frighten or sad*

    b. Amylin

    c. Aldosterone *- adrenal cortex - sodium/liver*

    d. Erythropoietin *cytokine made by kidneys*

14. *The resistance phase of Selye's general adaptation response is most supported by which hormone?*

    a. Progesterone

    (b.) Cortisol

    c. Noradrenaline

    d. Melatonin

    What is Selye gen adaptation RES

[handwritten notes at bottom:]
pituitary gland - endocrine gland gland secreats # of hormones regulate many bodily functions

hypothyroidism - inadequate levels of thyroid hormone - intolerance to cold, constipation, muscle aches

15. *Prolonged effects of lingering unresolved stress can predispose a person to type 2 diabetes since _____.*

    a. Cortisol supports a rise in blood levels of glucose, fatty acids, and amino acids
    b. Glucocorticoids reduce the activity of aldosterone, predisposing one to ketoacidosis
    c. Catecholamines inhibit sympathetic dominance pattern, resulting in excessive parasympathetic control over digestive processes
    d. Stress shuts down the production of adrenal cortex hormones, putting additional strain on the pancreas for glucose production

16. *What two endocrine glands secrete androgens?*

    a. Adrenals and pituitary
    b. Ovaries and thyroid
    c. Pineal and adrenals
    d. Testes and adrenals

    ↓ male hormone

17. *A client who is a marathon runner developed an inflammatory condition of the knee. As part of the treatment process, the client received an injection of corticosteroid into the area of the knee. The client wishes to have a deep massage of the area to reduce the pain. Why is this not appropriate?*

    a. The massage could decrease the inflammatory response and concentrate the medication at the injection site
    b. Deep massage increases the potential for localized inflammation and would disturb the action of the corticosteroid injection
    c. Deep massage would increase the tension of the muscles, causing instability, and inflammation would decrease
    d. Corticosteroids reduce inflammation and increase tissue repair; since massage increases the tendency for tissue repair, excessive scarring could result

Cortisol ~ same effects as as referred to as hydrocortisone

18. *A female client is experiencing some increase in coarse facial hair and acne. Which of the following hormones may be involved?*

    a. Androgen *male hormone*
    b. Estrogen
    c. Progesterone
    d. Endorphin

19. *Which of the following endocrine glands is most sensitive to light and dark cycles?*

    a. Adrenal
    b. Parathyroid
    c. Pineal
    d. Thymus

20. *Using the philosophy of the chakra system, a person practices compassion to self and others. Which endocrine gland is being supported?*

    a. Adrenal *~ kidney area   release a hoe that reg calcium &*
    b. Parathyroid *~ thyroid area   phosphor me.*
    c. Pineal
    d. Thymus *~ endocrine gland*

21. *Which of the following is the most common tissue hormone?*

    a. Prostaglandin *carbon-20 unsatured fattyacd*
    b. Cholecystokinin
    c. Atrial natriuretic factor
    d. Insulin-like growth factor

22. *In relationship to ancient chakra theory, if someone is concerned with not having enough money to pay bills, surviving a job change, and staying focused learning a new computer skill, which endocrine gland is likely to be affected?*

    a. Pituitary
    b. Thyroid
    c. Adrenal
    d. Pineal

 # 20 need chakra info ?

23. *A client has just experienced a job shift change from days to nights and is having difficulty adjusting the sleep pattern. The client indicates feeling disconnected and out of sorts. Which endocrine gland might initially be affected and which massage approach would be most beneficial?*

    a. Pineal gland; a massage that focuses on sympathetic stimulations with active participation by the client

    b. Adrenal glands; a massage that generates localized inflammatory areas, such as is found with direct pressure and friction on trigger points

    c. Thymus gland; a massage that uses sufficient pressure but pain-free compression and rhythmic gliding methods to support parasympathetic dominance

    d. Pineal gland; a massage that uses sufficient pressure but pain-free compression and rhythmic gliding methods to support parasympathetic dominance

Answers and Discussion

1. d
Application and concept identification
Rationale: Ancient healing traditions were based on observation through the centuries. While the technology was not available to validate theories by western scientific method, it is apparent that body anatomy and physiology were being observed. When one compares the chakra system to western theories of anatomy and physiology, the correlation with the endocrine system is understood.

2. c
Factual recall
Rationale: The question is a portion of the definition of a hormone.

3. a
Application and concept identification
Rationale: The question is asking for a relationship between the two systems of control in the body. The nervous system responds quickly to emergency situations, and then the endocrine system sustains the effect over a longer period of time.

4. a
Factual recall
Rationale: The correct answer describes a function of a hormone. The three incorrect answers are flawed and do not state true information in relationship to the question.

5. d
Factual recall
Rationale: The question is representative of terminology used for endocrine system pathology. Hyper means too much.

6. c
Factual recall
Rationale: The question describes a function of the hypothalamus. It would be necessary to know the function of the other structures listed to eliminate wrong answers and identify the correct answer.

7. b
Clinical reasoning/synthesis
Rationale: This question is representative of the type of case study found in relation to the content area—the endocrine system. Analysis of the question and possible answers leads to a correct decision. The facts presented by the question are: elderly client, slow tissue healing, gradual weight loss, and improvement in all areas after 3 months of weekly massage. The question asks for the justification of this outcome. The possible answers also list facts—some correct and others incorrect, some appropriate in relation to the question and others not. Research has shown that touch stimulates the hypothalamus. A function of the hypothalamus is to stimulate the pituitary to produce and release growth hormone, which would account for the benefits seen.

8. a
Factual recall
Rationale: The question asks for an understanding of the terms listed. The pituitary is the main source of tropic hormones.

9. b
Application and concept identification
Rationale: The question is asking for a connection between growth hormone function and behavior that supports it in the body. Only the correct answer supports growth hormone function. The other three possible answers indicate stress, which suppresses growth hormone function.

10. c
Application and concept identification
Rationale: The question is asking for a connection between hydrotherapy applications and pituitary hormones. The three incorrect answers are anterior pituitary hormones but have not been shown to be influenced by cold applications.

11. **b**
    Clinical reasoning/synthesis
    Rationale: This question is representative of the type of case study found in relation to the content area—the endocrine system. Analysis of the questions and possible answers would lead to a correct decision. The facts presented by the question are: middle-aged female, hypothyroid symptoms, increased stress and reduced ability to cope, no blood work done during the physical. The four answers list terminology that would have to be understood to identify the correct answer.

12. **c**
    Application and concept identification
    Rationale: The pancreatic pathology of type 2 diabetes is defined in the correct answer. The three incorrect answers provide misinformation. All of the terminology would have to be interpreted to find the incorrect word usage and identify the correct answer.

13. **a**
    Factual recall
    Rationale: The question is asking for the identification of the correct adrenal hormone that stimulates sympathetic function of the ANS. Epinephrine and aldosterone are adrenal hormones, but aldosterone is involved in water balance, so epinephrine is the correct answer.

14. **b**
    Application and concept identification
    Rationale: Selye's general adaptation response is described in many sources. This information is correlated with hormone function. Cortisol exerts a long-term effect on the body and therefore is more involved with resistance to stress.

15. **a**
    Application and concept identification
    Rationale: The question asks for a connection between long-term stress and the development of diabetes. The four possible answers provide explanations. Each of the terms in the answers needs to be defined to identify the correct answer. Only answer a makes the correct correlation.

16. **d**
    Factual recall
    Rationale: The terms in the question need to be defined to identify the correct answer. Androgens are gonadocorticoids and are produced both by the gonads and the adrenal glands.

17. **b**
    Clinical reasoning/synthesis
    Rationale: The facts provided in the question are: client is a runner, has an inflamed knee, received a steroid injection at the site, asks for deep massage to the area. The question indicates that this type of massage application is contraindicated, and the answer is to justify why this is so. Only answer b is a logical response. The other three answers present incorrect information. Massage of the site of a recent injection is contraindicated. Deep massage would tend to increase inflammation in the area. Corticosteroids decrease tissue repair processes.

18. **a**
    Application and concept identification
    Rationale: The question asks for a reason for the change in the condition of the client. An effect of androgen is increased facial hair and acne.

19. **c**
    Factual recall
    Rationale: The question is asking for an endocrine influence. The pineal gland is responsive to light and dark.

20. **d**
    Application and concept identification
    Rationale: The question is representative of how the ancient healing systems and Western thought are connected. It is necessary to understand the various chakra relationships to the endocrine glands to identify the correct answer. The thymus is correlated with the heart and spleen chakras.

21. **a**
    Factual recall
    Rationale: The four possible answers would need to be defined and identified to determine whether each is a tissue hormone and which is most common. Only prostaglandin is a tissue hormone.

22. **c**
    Application and concept identification
    Rationale: The question is representative of how the ancient healing systems and Western thought are connected. It is necessary to understand the various chakra relationships to the endocrine glands to identify the correct answer. The adrenal glands are correlated with the root chakra issues of survival.

23. **d**
    Clinical reasoning/synthesis
    Rationale: Three types of information are
    presented in the question and possible answers:
    the behavior change and result, what primary
    endocrine function is disrupted, and what
    massage intervention would support a return to
    homeostasis. All three areas must logically
    connect for a correct answer. Only the correct
    answer does this.

7

Skeletal System

Questions

1. Which of the following is not a function of bone?

   a. Storing minerals
   b. Producing blood cells
   c. Generating heat
   d. Storing lipids

2. A type of bone that develops in a tendon or joint capsule is a/n _____.

   a. Sesamoid bone *def*
   b. Piezo bone
   c. Articulation bone
   d. Compact bone

3. Which aspect of bone structure provides the elastic quality of bone?

   a. Inorganic mineral
   b. Organic material
   c. Trabeculae - *def*
   d. Endoskeleton

4. The main component of bone that has the piezoelectric quality is _____.

   a. Compact bone
   b. Cancellous bone
   c. Red marrow
   d. Collagen

5. The external connective tissue covering of bone is called the _____.

   a. Exoskeleton
   b. Endoskeleton
   c. Periosteum
   d. Endosteum

6. The continual changing of bone in response to functional demands is called _____.

   a. Remodeling
   b. Oppositional growth
   c. Haversian
   d. Articulation

7. Which type of bone contains trabeculae?

   a. Compact
   b. Cancellous
   c. Osteon
   d. Concentric

8. Which of the following bone types contains a diaphysis?

   a. Flat
   b. Irregular
   c. Long
   d. Sesamoid

9. *A young male client is experiencing a growth spurt. He complains that the bones in his legs ache. What is responsible for this phenomenon?*

   • a. Increased testosterone promotes long bone growth
   b. Increased estrogen promotes long bone growth
   c. Decreased estrogen supports long bone growth
   • d. Decreased testosterone promotes long bone growth

10. *Which of the following is a depression on a bone?*

   a. Condyle
   b. Fossa
   c. Line
   d. Tubercle

11. *Which of the following bones is located in the appendicular portion of the skeleton?*

   a. Ethmoid
   • b. Clavicle
   c. Sternum
   d. Coccyx

12. *Which suture joins the parietal bones and occipital bone?*

   a. Squamous
   b. Coronal
   c. Lambdoidal
   d. Sagittal

13. *Which of the following bones forms the structure of the nose?*

   a. Vomer
   b. Zygomatic
   c. Sphenoid
   d. Fontanelle

14. *What bone has a superior articular facet?*

   • a. Humerus
   b. Occipital
   c. Thoracic vertebrae
   d. Carpal

15. *Which of the following landmarks is located on the humerus?*

   a. Glenoid fossa
   b. Xiphoid process
   c. Radial styloid
   d. Olecranon fossa

16. *The coracoid process is located on which bone?*

   a. Scapula
   b. Sternum
   c. Femur
   d. Talus

17. *A client experienced an accident in which the trunk was thrust into extension. Which of the following structures might have been injured?*

   a. Deltoid ligament
   b. Anterior longitudinal ligament
   c. ASIS
   d. Linea aspera

18. *Which of the following is part of the pelvis?*

   a. Fovea
   b. Triquetrum
   c. Trochlear notch
   d. Acetabulum

19. *When one is palpating over the spine, the structure most prominently felt is _____.*

   a. Centrum
   b. Spinous process
   c. Annulus fibrosis
   d. Pedicle

20. *If an intervertebral disk rupture occurs, what is the possible outcome?*

   a. Narrowed disk space due to leakage of the nucleus pulposus
   b. Narrowed intervertebral space due to rupture of the fontanelle
   c. Impingement of the nerve from pressure exerted by the sella turcica
   d. Increased space in the foramen impinging on the spinal cord

21. When one is palpating the posterior cervical area, the fibrous structure felt is the _____.

    a. Kyphosis ligament
    b. Odontoid process
    c. Nuchal ligament
    d. Demifacets

22. The costal angle is located on which bone?

    a. Sternum
    b. Clavicle
    c. Atlas
    d. Rib

23. The foot typically contains how many bones?

    a. 31
    b. 26
    c. 12
    d. 22

24. A client complains of pain in the lower back. Observation indicates an excessive lumbar curve. This is called _____.

    a. Scoliosis
    b. Kyphosis
    c. Lordosis
    d. Talipes

25. A female client, age 67, has a history of smoking. This could indicate caution for compressive force used during massage for which reason?

    a. Osteonecrosis
    b. Osteomyelitis
    c. Osteochondritis dissecans
    d. Osteoporosis

26. A client complains of pain in the tibia. The client completed a marathon 24 hours before the massage session. What contraindication to massage may account for the pain?

    a. Stress fracture
    b. Compound fracture
    c. Dislocation
    d. Whiplash

Answers are on pages 52–53.

Answers and Discussion

1. **c**
   Factual recall
   Rationale: The question and possible answers identify bone function. Generating heat is a function of muscle, not bone.

2. **a**
   Factual recall
   Rationale: The question is the definition of a sesamoid bone.

3. **b**
   Factual recall
   Rationale: The question asks for the elastic component of bone provided by the organic material.

4. **d**
   Factual recall
   Rationale: The question asks for the piezo material of bone, which is collagen.

5. **c**
   Factual recall
   Rationale: The terms in the possible answers all need to be defined to answer the question. Periosteum is the external connective tissue covering of bone.

6. **a**
   Factual recall
   Rationale: The terms in the possible answers all need to be defined to answer the question. The question asks for the name of a bone function described as change in the bone in response to demand. This is remodeling.

7. **b**
   Factual recall
   Rationale: The terms in the question and possible answers all need to be defined to answer the question. Cancellous bone contains trabeculae.

8. **c**
   Factual recall
   Rationale: The terms in the question and possible answers all need to be defined to answer the question. Long bones contain a diaphysis.

9. **a**
   Application and concept identification
   Rationale: The question is asking for the connection between hormone effect on bone and symptoms of aching. Answer a explains why this could be happening. The other three answers present incorrect information. Estrogen and testosterone both produce long bone growth, but increasing estrogen levels, primarily in females, will also stop the growth. Since a male is described in the question, answer a is the correct answer.

10. **b**
    Factual recall
    Rationale: The question is asking for the identification of a bony landmark. All of the landmarks would need to be recognized to correctly answer this type of question.

11. **b**
    Factual recall
    Rationale: The question is asking for a classification of a bone by regions of the axial and appendicular skeleton. It is necessary to know what bones fall into these classifications to answer the question.

12. **c**
    Factual recall
    Rationale: This question is representative of a multitude of questions that could be written on the anatomy of bones. To answer the question it is necessary to correctly identify the location of the bones in the question and the suture that connects them.

13. **a**
    Factual recall
    Rationale: This question is representative of a multitude of questions that could be written on the anatomy of bones. To answer the question it is necessary to correctly identify the location of the bones in the possible answers provided.

14. **c**
    Factual recall
    Rationale: This question is representative of a multitude of questions that could be written on the anatomy of bones. To answer the question it is necessary to correctly identify which bone has the structure described in the question.

15. **d**
Factual recall
Rationale: This question is representative of a multitude of questions that could be written on the anatomy of bones. To answer the question it is necessary to correctly identify which bony landmark is located on the humerus.

16. **a**
Factual recall
Rationale: This question is representative of a multitude of questions that could be written on the anatomy of bones. To answer the question it is necessary to correctly identify which bone has a coracoid process. The scapula is the correct answer.

17. **b**
Application and concept identification
Rationale: This question is representative of many questions that could be written about movement and bone structure. This particular question asks for the connection between a structure connected with bone and an injury. If the trunk were put in exaggerated extension, the anterior longitudinal ligament could be overstretched.

18. **d**
Factual recall
Rationale: This question is representative of a multitude of questions that could be written on the anatomy of bones. To answer the question it is necessary to correctly identify which bone or bony structure is part of the pelvis. It is necessary to identify the location of all of the structures provided in the possible answers to identify acetabulum.

19. **b**
Factual recall
Rationale: This question is representative of a multitude of questions that could be written on the anatomy of bones. To answer the question it is necessary to correctly identify which bone or bony structure is part of the spine that can be easily palpated. It is necessary to identify the location of all of the structures provided in the possible answers to identify the spinous process.

20. **a**
Application and concept identification
Rationale: The question is asking what happens if the disk ruptures. The correct answer needs to be logical and contain correct terminology usage. All the terms would need to be defined to rule out wrong answers and identify the correct answer, a.

21. **c**
Factual recall
Rationale: This question is representative of a multitude of questions that could be written on the anatomy of bones. To answer the question it is necessary to correctly identify which bone or structure is part of the cervical spine that can be easily palpated. It is necessary to identify the location of all of the structures provided in the possible answers to identify the nuchal ligament. There is no structure called the kyphosis ligament. Incorrect use of terms is a common way to develop wrong answers.

22. **d**
Factual recall
Rationale: This question is representative of a multitude of questions that could be written on the anatomy of bones. To answer the question it is necessary to correctly identify which bone has a costal angle. It is necessary to identify the location of all of the structures provided in the possible answers to identify the ribs.

23. **b**
Factual recall
Rationale: This question is representative of a multitude of questions that could be written on the anatomy of bones.

24. **c**
Application and concept identification
Rationale: The question asks for the name of an excessive lumbar curve that may be responsible for low back pain. All the terms would need to be defined to identify the correct answer, lordosis.

25. **d**
Clinical reasoning/synthesis
Rationale: The facts in the question would help to identify the predisposition to the pathology of osteoporosis. The question also indicates that caution should be used during the massage since osteoporosis predisposes one to bone fracture.

26. **a**
Clinical reasoning/synthesis
Rationale: The facts in the question are: pain in the tibia, endurance running the day before. The possible answers indicate reasons for the pain. It is necessary to define the various pathologies of the skeletal system to rule out incorrect answers. The most logical answer is a stress fracture based on the history provided by the question.

8

Joints

Questions

1. *Joint function is a combined relationship between* _____.

   a. Bones and landmarks
   b. Stability and mobility
   c. Articulations and diarthroses
   d. Synovial fluid and pathologic range of motion

2. *The most complex joint design is likely to function in* _____.

   a. Stability
   b. Viscoelasticity
   c. Mobility
   d. Synarthrosis

3. *Principles and characteristics of joint design include all of the following* **except** _____.

   a. The design of a joint depends on its function
   b. The breakdown of any joint structure will affect the entire joint function
   c. Generally, stability must be achieved before mobility
   d. Most joints serve only one function, either stability or mobility

4. *What type of cartilage is found in joints that function primarily for mobility?*

   a. White fibrocartilage
   b. Hyaline cartilage
   c. Yellow fibrocartilage
   d. Synovial cartilage

5. *An important component of connective tissue that supports pliability is* _____.

   a. Water
   b. Synovial fluid
   c. Colloid
   d. Viscosity

6. *The viscoelasticity quality of connective tissue to modify in the direction of the force applied and then slowly return to the original state is called* _____.

   a. Plastic range
   b. Fibrous
   c. Creep
   d. Avulsion

7. *A client has been participating in a stretching program for over a year. Initially the program was very helpful, but during the last 3 months the program has become more aggressive and the client is complaining of joint pain. Which alteration in connective tissue may explain what has occurred?*

   a. The client has experienced a rupture in the connective tissue structures and has developed lax ligaments
   b. The client has exceeded the limits of the elastic range of the tissue, consistently deformed the tissue in the plastic range, and developed lax ligaments
   c. An avulsion failure of connective tissue has occurred, creating a decrease in mobility
   d. The tissue has become dehydrated, increasing creep tendency and contributing to stability provided by muscle contraction

8. *A client is complaining of a feeling of shortening and pulling in the area of the low back and sacroiliac joints. Assessment indicates decreased pliability in the connective tissue structures in this area. Which of the following massage applications is most appropriate to achieve an increase in short-term mobility without compromising stability or creating a remodeling process of the tissue?*

   a. Application of massage methods that slowly introduce creep, increasing pliability at the plastic range of the tissue

   b. Application of therapeutic inflammation coupled with stretching to exceed the plastic range of the tissue

   c. Application of elongation stretching to breach the plastic range of the tissue, creating inflammation to restore an appropriate creep pattern

   d. Application of abrupt bending of the connective tissue to support the increase in ligament laxity, thereby increasing mobility

9. *A client has been diagnosed with a hypermobile knee joint. Which of the following would be part of an appropriate treatment plan?*

   a. Extend the elastic range of connective tissue structures by altering the plastic range

   b. Elongate the plastic component of connective tissue in the direction of the shortening

   c. Restore pliability

   d. Manage muscle contraction around the joint using standard massage methods

10. *Which of the following joint types has the most limited mobility?*

    a. Syndesmosis
    b. Amphiarthrosis
    c. Cartilaginous
    d. Diarthrosis

11. *Which of the following is **not** a characteristic of a synovial joint?*

    a. A joint capsule formed of fibrous tissue
    b. Bones are separated by fibrocartilage
    c. Hyaline cartilage covers the joint surfaces
    d. Synovial fluid forms a lubricating film over the joint surfaces

12. *Which of the following joint structures is highly innervated and a source of sensory data concerning movement and position of a joint?*

    a. Stratum synovium
    b. Articular cartilage
    c. Stratum fibrosum
    d. Joint cavity

13. *A client is experiencing muscle spasms and reduced mobility around a shoulder joint that has a history of dislocation. Which of the following applications of massage would be best in assisting this client?*

    a. Increase the plastic range of the ligament structures and stretched tense muscles

    b. Use friction on tendons and ligaments, then incorporate a stretching program to increase flexibility

    c. Reduce muscle spasms to the point that mobility is supported but stability is not compromised

    d. Use massage methods and stretching to eliminate muscle spasms

14. *The accessory movements at a joint that describe how articulating surfaces move within the joint capsule and contribute to joint play are called* _____.

    a. Closed packed position
    b. Arthrokinematics
    c. Osteokinematics
    d. Range of motion

15. *Joints in which stability is reduced because of increased laxity of supportive ligaments will also have an increase in* _____.

    a. Joint play
    b. Hypomobility
    c. Muscle relaxation
    d. Plasma membrane

16. *The closed packed position of a joint can be described as _____.*

    a. The convex surface fitting minimally into the concave surface
    b. The position in which spin, roll, and slide most easily occur
    c. The position with the most joint play
    d. The convex surface fitting with maximal contact into the concave surface

17. *A client sprained the joint in one of the fingers. What is going to be the most comfortable position for the joint and why?*

    a. The closed packed position because this is the most stable position of the joint
    b. The loose packed position so that movement can most easily occur
    c. The least packed position to accommodate swelling
    d. The closed packed position to accommodate increased synovial fluid

18. *Which of the following describes a neurologic protective mechanism for normal joint function?*

    a. Anatomic range of motion
    b. Physiologic range of motion
    c. Pathologic range of motion
    d. Osteokinematics

19. *Which of the following joints has the least amount of bone structure creating the anatomic range of motion limits?*

    a. Elbow
    b. Hip
    c. Ankle
    d. Knee

20. *A client has a history of a broken wrist. The wrist was in a cast for an extended period of time because bone repair was slower than normal. The client is now experiencing a decrease in range of motion of the wrist. What might be the cause?*

    a. Hypomobility due to contracture
    b. Hypomobility due to reduced muscle tension
    c. Hypermobility due to increased muscle tension
    d. Hypomobility due to increased anatomic range of motion

21. *During the massage session passive joint movement is used for assessing the range of motion of the arm during circumduction. Which of the following best describes the action used during this process?*

    a. Bending movement that decreased the angle of a joint
    b. Movement of arm medially toward the midline of the body
    c. Twisting and turning of a bone on its own axis
    d. Combined movements of flexion, extension, abduction, adduction to create a cone shape

22. *Before the massage session begins and during the initial physical assessment, active joint movement is used to assess the range of motion of the foot. Which term is most correct to use to describe a portion of this activity?*

    a. Pronation
    b. Supination
    c. Eversion
    d. Opposition

23. *The term used to describe the movement of the scapula toward the spine is _____.*

    a. Rotation
    b. Retraction
    c. Protraction
    d. Elevation

24. *During assessment you want the client to externally rotate the hip. What instructions would you give the client?*

    a. Please move your leg so that you cross it over the other leg at the ankles
    b. Please straighten your legs and turn the entire leg so that you point your toes toward each other
    c. Please straighten your legs and turn the entire leg so that you point your toes away from each other
    d. Please bring your knee toward your chest

Answers are on pages 61–64.

25. A ball-and-socket joint is also considered a
_____.

    a. Pivot joint
    b. Biaxial joint
    c. Gliding joint
    d. Multiaxial joint

26. The name of the association between joints as
they function in relationship to each other is
called _____.

    a. Joint play
    b. Osteokinematics
    c. Kinematic chains
    d. Diarthrosis

27. The function of joints that is often going to result
in a compensation pattern in one joint if there is
a change in function in another joint is called the
_____.

    a. Closed kinematic chain
    b. Open kinematic chain
    c. Loose packed kinematic chain
    d. Closed packed kinematic chain

28. The two articulating bones of the temporomandibular joint are the _____.

    a. Temporal and maxilla
    b. Mandible and maxilla
    c. Mandible and temporal
    d. Temporal and zygomatic

29. The glenohumeral joint has extensive mobility
because _____.

    a. It has range-of-motion limits provided
    primarily by soft tissue
    b. Physiologic limits to range of motion provide
    for a loose fit between the humerus and the
    clavicle
    c. Of its biaxial joint structure, which allows
    movement in three planes
    d. Of the ball-and-socket joint structure, which
    allows movement only in two planes

30. Which is a movement allowed at the sternoclavicular joint?

    a. Flexion
    b. Rotation
    c. Inversion
    d. Extension

31. Should there be an injury to the sternoclavicular
joint that limits its range of motion, what other
structure will be affected?

    a. Radius
    b. Olecranon
    c. Scapula
    d. Deltoid ligament

32. The coracoclavicular ligament is part of what
joint?

    a. Glenohumeral
    b. Temporomandibular
    c. Sternoclavicular
    d. Acromioclavicular

33. Which of the following joints is responsible for
pronation and supination?

    a. Ulnar-humeral
    b. Radioulnar
    c. Radiohumeral
    d. Radiocarpal

34. A wrist movement is greatest in flexion and
extension because _____.

    a. The joint capsule is loose in the superior and
    inferior directions
    b. The joint type is a hinge joint
    c. The joint capsule is loose laterally and
    medially
    d. The radiocarpal joint forms a direct contact
    between the ulna and the carpal bones

35. The joint where the fingers join the body of the
hand is called the _____.

    a. Distal interphalangeal joint
    b. Proximal interphalangeal joint
    c. Metacarpophalangeal joint
    d. Intercarpal joint

36. *The articulating bones of the sacroiliac joint are the _____.*
    a. Sacrum and ischium
    b. Sacrum and iliac
    c. Sacrum and acetabulum
    d. Sacrum and pubis

37. *Which of the following joints has no direct muscle action but is responsible for helping the vertebral column to remain relatively still during walking?*
    a. Symphysis pubis
    b. Sacral lumbar
    c. Labrum
    d. Sacroiliac

38. *The loose packed position of the hip joint is ____.*
    a. Flexion, abduction, and lateral rotation
    b. Extension, adduction, and medial rotation
    c. Flexion, adduction, and lateral rotation
    d. Extension, abduction, and lateral rotation

39. *If the leg is fixed and does not move and the pelvis moves forward into anteversion, what is the result?*
    a. Increased kyphosis
    b. Increased lordosis
    c. Decreased lordosis
    d. Decreased scoliosis

40. *The most stable position of the knee joint is _____.*
    a. In slight flexion
    b. In full hyperextension
    c. In locked extension
    d. In locked flexion

41. *A client was playing football when tackled. Pressure was put on the lateral side of the left knee. Which ligament would receive the most extension strain?*
    a. Lateral collateral
    b. Medial collateral
    c. Posterior cruciate
    d. Posterior meniscofemoral

42. *Which fibrocartilaginous structure allows for more surface contact of the femur on the tibia?*
    a. Cruciates
    b. Labrum
    c. Patella
    d. Menisci

43. *The most stable position of the ankle joint is _____.*
    a. Plantar flexion
    b. Plantar rotation
    c. Full dorsiflexion
    d. Rotated eversion

44. *A client continues to sprain the ankles. You notice that the client wears boots with a 2-inch heel. How would this contribute to injury potential?*
    a. The heel positions the ankle in dorsiflexion, making the ankle joint less stable
    b. The heel positions the ankle in plantar flexion, making the ankle joint less stable
    c. The weight is shifted to the ball of the foot, creating an open kinematic chain
    d. The inferior tibiofibular joint is extended when the heel is raised and creates instability

45. *Which of the following joints allows rotation as a motion pattern?*
    a. Atlantooccipital
    b. Atlantoaxial
    c. Intervertebral
    d. Costovertebral

46. *Which movement of the vertebral joints is most stabilized by the anterior longitudinal ligament?*
    a. Extension
    b. Flexion
    c. Rotation
    d. Lateral flexion

Answers are on pages 61–64.

47. *During the history interview a client reports experiencing a disk herniation posterior in the low back. Which type of injury and what likely location would be indicated?*

    a. Extension injury at the sacrolumbar junction
    b. Flexion injury at T-12
    c. Flexion injury at the lumbosacral junction
    d. Extension injury at the thoracolumbar junction

48. *Which two joints are most active during breathing?*

    a. Intervertebral and costovertebral
    b. Vertebral arch and chondrosternal
    c. Costochondral and intervertebral
    d. Costovertebral and costochondral

49. *What is the action of the ribs during inspiration?*

    a. Ribs lowered
    b. Ribs raised
    c. Ribs protracted
    d. Ribs retracted

50. *Which of the following pathologic conditions of the joints responds most positively to massage?*

    a. Dislocation
    b. Rheumatoid arthritis
    c. Lateral epicondylitis
    d. Kyphosis

51. *A client has received a diagnosis of degenerative joint disease. Conservative treatment measures are indicated. Which of the following treatment plans is most appropriate?*

    a. Bed rest with over-the-counter antiinflammatory medication
    b. Cortisone injections and moderate exercise
    c. Ice, regular intense exercise, and connective tissue massage
    d. Ice, moderate exercise, general massage, and counterirritation ointments

52. *A client has a sore shoulder from a work-related repetitive overuse injury. The client has held the shoulder in the least packed position both with a sling and through muscle holding for over 3 months. Now the client is experiencing reduced range of motion. Which of the following is most helped by massage?*

    a. Protective muscle splinting that has developed shortened connective tissue patterns
    b. Nerve impingement
    c. Arthritis
    d. Adhesive capsulitis

Answers and Discussion

1. **b**
Application and concept identification
Rationale: Function of joints is based on stability and mobility. Bones, landmarks, articulations, diarthroses, and synovial fluid do not describe function.

2. **c**
Factual recall
Rationale: The function of simple joint design is stability and that of complex joint design is mobility.

3. **d**
Factual recall
Rationale: The question is representative of the type that asks for identification of only the wrong answer. These types of questions need to be carefully read. In this question answer d is the correct choice since the other possible answers do describe characteristics of joint design. Many joints serve a dual function of stability and mobility.

4. **b**
Factual recall
Rationale: The terminology needs to be defined. Hyaline cartilage is found at the ends of bone in synovial joints.

5. **a**
Factual recall
Rationale: A major component of ground substance is water.

6. **c**
Factual recall
Rationale: The terms need to be defined to understand the question and identify the correct answer. The question is the definition of creep.

7. **b**
Clinical reasoning/synthesis
Rationale: The facts presented in the question are: 1-year stretching program that was initially beneficial and increased intensity of the program in the last 3 months, resulting in joint pain. The question wants to know why this is the outcome based on changes in connective tissue structure. Each of the answers provides an explanation, but the three wrong answers present flawed data. Analysis is necessary to identify errors and find the correct answer. Only answer b presents correct information in relation to the facts of the question and indicates a logical explanation for the decrease in joint stability and development of joint pain.

8. **a**
Clinical reasoning/ synthesis
Rationale: The case study format presents the following facts: sensation of shortening in the lumbosacral area, confirmed by assessment revealing decreased mobility of the tissue in the area. Next limits are put on the type of intervention allowed. The correct answer needs to stay within these limits yet address the problem. Knowledge of the physiologic effects of massage methods on connective tissue physiology is necessary to correctly analyze for the appropriate answer. The three incorrect answers are not logical and would present cautions with their use. Only answer a presents a treatment plan that is cautious yet effective.

9. **d**
Clinical reasoning/synthesis
Rationale: The facts presented by the question are limited to information about a hypermobile knee joint. Safe application of massage methods is always a priority. The three wrong answers would all further increase the hypermobility; therefore, answer d is the most logical approach since the protective and compensatory muscle contraction is not eliminated but instead managed.

10. **a**
Factual recall
Rationale: Defining the terminology is necessary to answer the question.

11. **b**
Factual recall
Rationale: This is an example of identification of the incorrect statement as the answer of choice. Always read this type of question carefully. Synovial joints are freely movable, and fibrocartilage is found in synarthrodial joints.

12. **c**
Factual recall
Rationale: Defining the terms is necessary to answer the question.

13. **c**

    Clinical reasoning/synthesis
    Rationale: The facts presented by the question are information about multiple dislocations of a shoulder joint that now has reduced mobility and muscle spasms. Safe application of massage methods is always a priority. The three wrong answers would all further increase the underlying hypermobility. Answer c is the most logical approach since the protective and compensatory muscle contraction is not eliminated but instead managed.

14. **b**

    Factual recall
    Rationale: The question is the definition of arthrokinematics.

15. **a**

    Application and concept identification
    Rationale: The concepts presented in the question are stability and laxity, and in the answers they are joint play, hypomobility, and muscle relaxation. The term plasma membrane refers to cellular structure. The question wants to know what happens when lax ligaments reduce stability, and the answer is joint play increases.

16. **d**

    Factual recall
    Rationale: The correct answer defines the closed packed position of a joint.

17. **c**

    Application and concept identification
    Rationale: The question asks why the least packed position is the most comfortable when a joint is injured.

18. **b**

    Factual recall
    Rationale: The question is the definition of physiologic range of motion.

19. **d**

    Factual recall
    Rationale: The question asks for information about joint structure. This question represents the type of question in which an understanding of how joints are designed is necessary to answer the question. The anatomic limits of motion of the knee are primarily provided by soft tissue, such as the joint capsule and ligaments, instead of bone, as found in the elbow and hip. The ankle is similar to the knee but held more stable by the bone structure.

20. **a**

    Clinical reasoning/synthesis
    Rationale: The case study question structure requires an analysis of the data provided in the question and possible answers. The facts are: a broken wrist, extended period of joint immobility while in a cast, and current limited range of motion of the wrist. The correct answer would explain why this has occurred. The condition described is hypomobility, so answer c can be eliminated. Muscles atrophy when immobile, so answer b is eliminated. Answer d is an incorrect use of terminology. The only answer left is answer a, which would be the probable outcome.

21. **d**

    Application and concept identification
    Rationale: The question asks for the connection between a massage method (passive range of motion) and how the method would be implemented. Only answer d correctly describes circumduction.

22. **c**

    Factual recall
    Rationale: The terms in the possible answers need to be defined to identify eversion as a movement of the foot.

23. **b**

    Factual recall
    Rationale: The terms in the possible answers need to be defined to identify scapular retraction.

24. **c**

    Application and concept identification
    Rationale: The question is asking for how correct information is transmitted to a client so that a joint movement can be performed for either assessment or intervention. The action described by the correct answer needs to result in the external rotation of the hip. Only answer c is correct.

25. **d**

    Factual recall
    Rationale: The terms need to be defined to identify the correct answer.

26. **c**

    Factual recall
    Rationale: The question is the definition of kinematic chains.

27. **a**
    Factual recall
    Rationale: The question describes the outcome of functional change in closed kinematic chains. The terminology is used incorrectly in possible answers c and d. This is often a strategy for creating incorrect answers.

28. **c**
    Factual recall
    Rationale: This question is representative of many possible questions relating to joint anatomy. It is necessary to identify the two correct articulating bones of the joint to correctly answer the question.

29. **a**
    Factual recall
    Rationale: This question is representative of many possible questions relating to joint anatomy. It is necessary to identify the correct structural design of the joint to answer the question.

30. **b**
    Factual recall
    Rationale: This question is representative of many possible questions relating to joint function. It is necessary to identify the correct structural design of the joint to answer the question.

31. **c**
    Application and concept identification
    Rationale: The question is asking for the relationship between two joints, the sternoclavicular joint and the scapula.

32. **d**
    Factual recall
    Rationale: This question is representative of many possible questions relating to joint anatomy. It is necessary to identify the correct structural design of the joint to answer the question.

33. **b**
    Factual recall
    Rationale: This question is representative of many possible questions relating to joint function. It is necessary to identify the correct structural design and movement pattern of the joint to answer the question.

34. **a**
    Factual recall
    Rationale: This question is representative of many possible questions relating to joint anatomy. It is necessary to identify the correct structural design of the joint to answer the question. The question requires understanding of the terminology to identify the correct answer.

35. **c**
    Factual recall
    Rationale: This question is representative of many possible questions relating to joint anatomy. It is necessary to identify the correct articulating bones of the joint to answer the question. The question requires understanding of the terminology to identify the correct answer.

36. **b**
    Factual recall
    Rationale: This question is representative of many possible questions relating to joint anatomy. It is necessary to identify the correct articulating bones of the joint to answer the question. The question requires understanding of the terminology to identify the correct answer.

37. **d**
    Factual recall
    Rationale: This question is representative of many possible questions relating to joint function. It is necessary to identify the correct structural design of the joint to answer the question. The question requires understanding of the terminology to identify the correct answer.

38. **a**
    Application and concept identification
    Rationale: This question is representative of many possible questions relating to joint function. It is necessary to identify the correct movement of the joint into the loose packed position to answer the question. The question requires understanding of the terminology to identify the correct answer.

39. **b**
    Application and concept identification
    Rationale: This question is representative of many possible questions relating to joint movement patterns. It is necessary to identify the correct result in response to anteversion to answer the question. The question requires understanding of the terminology to identify the correct answer.

40. **c**
    Application and concept identification
    Rationale: This question is representative of
    many possible questions relating to joint
    function. It is necessary to identify the most
    stable position of the knee to answer the
    question. The question requires understanding
    of the terminology to identify the correct answer.

41. **b**
    Application and concept identification
    Rationale: This question is representative of
    many possible questions relating to joint
    anatomy in response to trauma. It is necessary to
    identify the correct outcome of the trauma to
    answer the question. In this instance the medial
    ligament would be pushed into extension and
    the damage would occur. The question requires
    understanding of the terminology to identify the
    correct answer.

42. **d**
    Factual recall
    Rationale: The question describes the function of
    the menisci.

43. **c**
    Factual recall
    Rationale: The most stable position is full
    dorsiflexion.

44. **b**
    Application and concept identification
    Rationale: The question asks for an explanation
    as to why the heel would increase potential for
    sprained ankle. The heel puts the ankle into
    plantar flexion, which is a less stable position for
    the ankle, predisposing to ankle sprains.

45. **b**
    Factual recall
    Rationale: Knowledge about the range of motion
    allowed at the listed joints is necessary to answer
    the question.

46. **a**
    Application and concept identification
    Rationale: The connection between the location
    of the anterior longitudinal ligament and its
    function in relation to the vertebral joints is
    required to answer the question. This ligament
    stabilizes against trunk extension.

47. **c**
    Clinical reasoning/synthesis
    Rationale: The facts presented in the question
    indicate that the disk bulged posteriorly, which
    would be the result of a flexion injury. The most
    common location in the lower back is at the
    lumbosacral junction.

48. **d**
    Factual recall
    Rationale: Knowledge about the range of motion
    allowed at the listed joints is necessary to answer
    the question.

49. **b**
    Factual recall
    Rationale: Recall of rib motion during breathing
    in is required to answer the question. The ribs
    are raised during inspiration.

50. **c**
    Application and concept identification
    Rationale: The pathologies listed need to be
    defined and then benefits of massage correlated
    with possible outcomes. Dislocation is contrain-
    dicated. Rheumatoid arthritis has a limited
    response to massage and requires caution.
    Kyphosis is structural. Only answer c is correct.

51. **d**
    Clinical reasoning/synthesis
    Rationale: The question provides the following
    fact: the client has degenerative joint disease.
    The textbook provides additional information
    about this disorder. The question also places
    cautions on treatment, indicating use of
    conservative measures. The correct treatment
    plan would need to address both the condition
    and the cautions. Bed rest is not indicated nor is
    cortisone injection used for conservative treat-
    ment. Intense exercise and connective tissue
    massage are too aggressive. Answer d presents
    the best plan.

52. **a**
    Clinical reasoning/synthesis
    Rationale: The facts from the question are:
    repetitive strain injury, long-term decreased
    mobility, and reduced range of motion. Of the
    possible reasons for the reduced range of
    motion, massage would best reverse muscle and
    connective tissue pathology.

9

Muscles

Questions

1. Muscle uses which of the following to produce mechanical energy to exert force?

   a. Myoglobin
   b. Adenosine triphosphate
   c. Perimysium
   d. Cholecystokinin

2. A client complains of fatigue and muscle soreness after attempting to push a car that was stuck. Which of the follow best describes this action?

   a. No movement was produced, so static force was generated
   b. Dynamic force was used since the car did not move
   c. Static force produced movement and energy expenditure
   d. Since the car did not move, little energy was expended

3. During assessment the massage professional realizes that a client has extremely mobile joints. Which muscle functions would seem to be impaired?

   a. Produce movement
   b. Generate heat
   c. Maintain posture
   d. Stabilize joints

4. When a joint flexes, the muscles producing the action will shorten. Which of the functional characteristics of muscles is being described?

   a. Excitability
   b. Contractility
   c. Extensibility
   d. Elasticity

5. The structural units of contraction in skeletal muscle fibers are _____.

   a. Myoglobin
   b. Myofibril
   c. Sarcomeres
   d. Fascicle

6. The attachment of myosin to cross-bridges on actin requires _____.

   a. Calcium
   b. Maximal stimulus
   c. Endomysium
   d. Potassium

7. Delicate and precise movements such as found with the eye muscles are possible because _____.

   a. Multiple sensory neurons innervate the muscles
   b. Large motor units exist in the muscle
   c. The muscle fibers in a motor unit are clustered together
   d. A motor unit consists of a few muscle fibers

8. Anatomically there is a strong correlation between the location of motor points, acupuncture points, and _____.

   a. Motor end plates
   b. Tendons
   c. Trigger points
   d. Mitotic units

9. The nature of muscles to maintain a certain amount of tautness is called _____.

   a. Threshold stimulus
   b. Muscle tone
   c. Treppe
   d. All-or-none response

10. A client was a sprinter in high school track and was very effective during short and quick runs. Now 10 years later the client is complaining of lacking the endurance to run 5 miles as part of a fitness program. The client is in good physical condition with no apparent reason for the difficulties. Which of the following offers the most plausible explanation for the client's condition?

    a. The person has an abundance of slow twitch fibers in relationship to fast twitch fibers
    b. The person has an increased ability to manage oxygen debt
    c. The person's legs have a genetic tendency toward a makeup of more white anaerobic fibers
    d. The person has increased slow twitch fibers in the postural muscles

11. A client is complaining of tender areas in the postural muscles along the spine. Assessment indicates a series of trigger points in these muscles. The massage professional must determine how much compressive force to apply to the trigger points and how long to hold the contraction. Which of the following will affect this decision?

    a. These muscles contain more slow twitch red fiber that are fatigue resistant
    b. These muscles are prone to oxygen debt
    c. These muscles have an abundance of fast twitch and intermediate fibers
    d. These muscles require a maximal stimulus in order to respond to treatment

12. Vascular structures in muscles are _____.

    a. Limited to the muscular aponeurosis
    b. Abundant and designed to accommodate stretch
    c. Found mainly in the epimysium
    d. Abundant within the ligament structures

13. The connective tissue aspect of muscles is _____.

    a. The active contractile unit
    b. The main heat-producing structure
    c. Responsive to ATP
    d. Inseparable and continuous with muscle fibers

14. Intermuscular septa are formed primarily from _____.

    a. Deep fascia
    b. Epimysium
    c. Perimysium
    d. Endomysium

15. A client complains of a sensation of thickness and stiffness in the myofascial structures of the body. Slow sustained stretching provides the most benefit. What is the most plausible reason for this effect?

    a. The neuromuscular unit is deprived of calcium, allowing the actin and myosin to disengage
    b. The viscous nature of connective tissue responds to this method by becoming more plastic
    c. The colloid connective tissue ground substance decreases water binding with these methods
    d. The compression against the capillaries increases blood flow

16. *Two clients describe accidents in which the muscles of their upper thigh were cut and now healed. Client A has a mobile scar with near normal function. Client B has tissue rigidity and reduced movement. What is the most plausible explanation?*

    a. Client A limited exercise and kept the area tightly wrapped during the healing process
    b. Client B had more satellite cell activity during healing, causing increased scar tissue
    c. Client A exercised during healing to stimulate satellite cells
    d. Client B experienced increased circulation and reduced adhesions

17. *The proximal attachment of a muscle is also known as the _____.*

    a. Origin
    b. Insertion
    c. Direct attachment
    d. Indirect attachment

18. *A client is complaining of pain when straightening the elbow. Palpation of the triceps at the musculotendinous junction indicates more tenderness at the insertion when the muscle is activated. What is the most likely reason for this?*

    a. The insertion is the fixed attachment and would be more tender during movement.
    b. The insertion is the proximal attachment and is straining at the intermuscular septa
    c. The belly of the muscle located at the insertion is highly innervated
    d. The insertion is the more movable attachment so it would produce more tenderness upon motion

19. *If a strong and sustained contraction without extensive movement is required, which of the following muscle shapes provides the best design?*

    a. Parallel
    b. Pennate
    c. Circular
    d. Convergent

20. *A client is experiencing a limitation in range of motion of the hip into abduction. Assessment indicates shortening and tension in the adductor group of muscles. Which of the following is the most likely source of the limited range of motion?*

    a. Agonists
    b. Synergists
    c. Antagonists
    d. Fixators

21. *The ability to execute a coordinated and accurate pattern of movement requires cooperation among various muscle groups called _____.*

    a. Myotatic units
    b. Stretch reflex
    c. Tendon reflex
    d. Inhibition

22. *The polysynaptic reflex that coordinates muscle action on both sides of the body is the _____.*

    a. Stretch reflex
    b. Flexor reflex
    c. Tendon reflex
    d. Fixator reflex

23. *A client unexpectedly lifted a box that was much too heavy. Now the client is experiencing residual weakness in the biceps and brachialis muscles and tension in the triceps muscle group. Which of the following reflexes best explains this situation?*

    a. Stretch reflex
    b. Tendon reflex
    c. Withdrawal reflex
    d. Crossed extensor reflex

24. *Which of the following muscle types has the ability to contract in such a way as to produce peristalsis?*

    a. Cardiac
    b. Circular
    c. Smooth
    d. Pennate

Answers are on pages 72–77.

25. *A client is complaining of a headache in the eye, ear, and scalp, especially above the ear. Assessment identifies a trigger point in which of the following muscles?*

    a. Orbicularis oculi
    b. Buccinator
    c. Risorius
    d. Occipitofrontalis

26. *Which of the following is a muscle of mastication?*

    a. Platysma
    b. Lateral pterygoid
    c. Digastric
    d. Zygomaticus major

27. *The muscles of the anterior triangle of the neck as defined by the sternocleidomastoid have a primary function of _____.*

    a. Assisting in swallowing
    b. Cervical extension
    c. Stabilization of capital rotation
    d. Neck flexion

28. *Compression by which of the following muscle groups against the brachial nerve plexus often refers pain to the pectoralis, to the rhomboid area, and into the arm and hand?*

    a. Splenius capitis and cervicis
    b. Erector spinae group
    c. Scalene group
    d. Infrahyoid group

29. *The abdominals and psoas muscles are the major antagonists for which of the following muscles?*

    a. Splenius capitis
    b. Longissimus thoracis
    c. Intertransversarii thoracis
    d. Serratus posterior

30. *A client complains of difficulty achieving a full and deep breath. Assessments indicate no problems with exhalation. There is a restriction with the lifting of the ribs during inhalation. Which muscle that lifts the ribs may be involved?*

    a. Diaphragm
    b. Serratus posterior inferior
    c. Internal intercostals
    d. External intercostals

31. *A client complains of low back pain that increases with coughing. Assessment indicates tenderness in the deep lumbar area with referred pain to the gluteal area, particularly around the sacroiliac joint. Which muscle is likely to be involved?*

    a. Quadratus lumborum
    b. Iliacus
    c. Semispinalis
    d. Psoas minor

32. *Which of the following muscles has its origin at the crest of the pubis and pubic symphysis and insertion at the cartilage of the fifth, sixth, and seventh ribs and at the xiphoid process?*

    a. Pyramidalis
    b. External oblique
    c. Rectus abdominis
    d. Transversus abdominis

33. *Which of the following muscles would be innervated by the perineal division of the pudendal nerve?*

    a. Levator ani
    b. Cremaster
    c. Longus colli
    d. Levator labii inferioris

34. *Which of the following muscles of scapular stabilization contains three distinct parts with distinct functions, allowing the muscle to be an antagonist to itself?*

    a. Serratus anterior
    b. Trapezius
    c. Pectoralis minor
    d. Rhomboid major

35. *Assessment indicates that a client has the left scapular area rounded forward and protracted. Which of the following muscles are likely to be tense and shortened?*

    a. Trapezius and rhomboid minor
    b. Levator scapula and supraspinatus
    c. Pectoralis minor and serratus anterior
    d. Teres minor and infraspinatus

36. *Assessment indicates that a client has bilateral medially rotated humerus. The subscapularis muscles are tight and short and contain trigger points. Which of the following muscles is likely to be inhibited?*

    a. Anterior deltoid
    b. Pectoralis major
    c. Teres major
    d. Infraspinatus

37. *A client is having difficulty raising the arm into a position to comb the hair. Which of the following muscles is likely to be tight and short?*

    a. Coracobrachialis
    b. Biceps brachii
    c. Latissimus dorsi
    d. Teres minor

38. *Which muscle is attached as follows: distal half of the anterior surface of the humerus, medial and lateral intermuscular septa, and coronoid process and tuberosity of the ulna?*

    a. Brachioradialis
    b. Pronator teres
    c. Supinator
    d. Brachialis

39. *Which of the following muscles is synergistic to the triceps?*

    a. Supinator
    b. Pronator quadratus
    c. Anconeus
    d. Pronator teres

40. *A client has been working on a project that required gripping a hammer for an extended period. Now the client is complaining of weakness when attempting to extend the wrist. Which of the following is the most likely explanation?*

    a. The flexor muscle group of the hand and wrist increased tone levels, resulting in inhibition of the extensor group of muscles in the forearm
    b. The flexor digitorum superficialis and profundus are weak from fatigue, so the wrist extensors have been facilitated
    c. The deep layer of the posterior wrist extensor group is antagonistic to the superficial layer of this same muscle group, resulting in weakness in the wrist extensors
    d. The flexor carpi ulnaris and the extensor carpi ulnaris are both in spasm, resulting in inhibition of the abductor pollicis longus

41. *Which of the following muscles is located in the thenar eminence?*

    a. Opponens digiti minimi
    b. Opponens pollicis
    c. Lumbricales
    d. Dorsal interosseus

42. *Which of the following muscles extends, laterally rotates the hip joint with lower fibers, assists in adduction of the hip with the femur fixed, and assists in extension of the trunk?*

    a. Gluteus medius
    b. Gluteus minimus
    c. Gluteus maximus
    d. Tensor fasciae latae

43. *When considering the layering of muscles from superficial to deep, which of the following is the deepest?*

    a. Gluteus medius
    b. Gluteus minimus
    c. Gluteus maximus
    d. Piriformis

Answers are on pages 72–77.

44. *Observation and assessment of a client indicate that the left leg is externally (laterally) rotated. Which of the following muscles may be tense and shortened?*

    a. Tensor fasciae latae
    b. Gemellus superior
    c. Gracilis
    d. Pectineus

45. *Which of the following pairs of muscles are synergistic with each other?*

    a. Biceps femoris and gluteus maximus
    b. Adductor brevis and gluteus medius
    c. Semimembranosus and obturator externus
    d. Piriformis and semitendinosus

46. *If the legs are fixed, which of the following is a flexor of the hip and also assists in flexion of the torso to the thigh?*

    a. Vastus lateralis
    b. Vastus medialis
    c. Sartorius
    d. Semitendinosus

47. *A client complains of difficulty extending the knee. Which group of muscles is likely to be tense and short?*

    a. Adductor group
    b. Quadriceps femoris group
    c. Anterior leg group
    d. Hamstring group

48. *When beginning flexion, a client feels a "catch" sensation in the back of the knee. The doctor does not find any problem with the joint and indicates that it is a muscular problem. Which muscle is likely to be involved?*

    a. Peroneus brevis
    b. Tibialis posterior
    c. Popliteus
    d. Peroneus longus

49. *Which muscles are most responsible for dorsiflexion?*

    a. Anterior leg muscles
    b. Posterior leg muscles
    c. Lateral leg muscles
    d. Medial leg muscles

50. *A dancer is finding it difficult to sustain movement requiring him to be on his toes. Which muscle may be inhibited?*

    a. Plantar interossei
    b. Soleus
    c. Extensor digitorum
    d. Peroneus tertius

51. *Which of the following muscles plantar flexes the ankle and assists with knee flexion?*

    a. Tibialis posterior
    b. Tibialis anterior
    c. Peroneus longus
    d. Plantaris

52. *If the gastrocnemius is tight and short, which of the following muscles is likely to be inhibited?*

    a. Soleus
    b. Tibialis anterior
    c. Flexor hallucis longus
    d. Flexor digitorum longus

53. *Which of the following muscles has its attachment on the larger or great toe?*

    a. Flexor digitorum brevis
    b. Quadratus plantae
    c. Flexor hallucis brevis
    d. Abductor digiti minimi

54. *A client's job requires her to perform the same repetitive lift and hand squeeze task. She has been doing this job for 8 months. In the beginning, her arms were sore and a bit swollen but that went away. In the past 3 months, the pain and tension in the arms have returned and begun to increase. Which of the following best describes the client's current condition?*

    a. Chain reaction in myotatic units has occurred
    b. Pain increases tension or spasm, which increases pain
    c. Joint restriction and fascial shortening decrease mobility
    d. Generalized fatigue has developed from an interrupted sleep pattern

55. *Which of the following medications would likely be prescribed for tendinitis?*

    a. Antibiotic
    b. Muscle relaxant
    c. Anticoagulant
    d. Antiinflammatory

56. *A client is taking an over-the-counter analgesic. What concern would the massage professional have while providing massage?*

    a. Feedback mechanisms for pain will be altered
    b. Blood pressure may fall dangerously low
    c. The infection may be spread
    d. Inflammation may be increased

57. *Which of the following conditions is most likely to benefit directly from a nonspecific general massage session?*

    a. Contusion
    b. Anterior compartment syndrome
    c. Muscle tension headache
    d. Spasticity

58. *Which of the following conditions presents regional contraindications for massage as long as physician approval has been obtained?*

    a. Postpolio syndrome
    b. Myositis ossificans
    c. Muscular dystrophy
    d. Myasthenia gravis

59. *A client with fibromyalgia has been referred from the physician for massage. A treatment plan has been requested for approval before treatment begins. Which of the following would be the best approach?*

    a. General massage with active assisted joint movement and stretching
    b. General massage with friction methods to active tender points
    c. Localized massage to the feet and ischemic compression to active trigger points
    d. General massage to support restorative sleep and symptomatic pain management

Answers are on pages 72–77.

Answers and Discussion

1. **b**
   Factual recall
   Rationale: All the possible answers would need to be defined to identify adenosine triphosphate (ATP) as the correct answer.

2. **a**
   Application and concept identification
   Rationale: The question is asking for the connection among an action (pushing a car), the result (fatigue and muscle soreness), and the best description for the action. Generating static force expends energy with no result in movement.

3. **d**
   Application and concept identification
   Rationale: Assessment identifies hypermobile joints. The correct answer explains the role of muscles in joint stability.

4. **b**
   Factual recall
   Rationale: The terms listed as possible answers need to be defined to answer the question.

5. **c**
   Factual recall
   Rationale: The terms listed as possible answers need to be defined to answer the question.

6. **a**
   Factual recall
   Rationale: The terms in the question and listed as possible answers need to be defined to answer the question.

7. **d**
   Factual recall
   Rationale: The questions and possible answers describe a physiologic process in terms of muscle contractile ability and control based on the number of muscle fibers per motor unit. The fewer the fibers, the more precise the movement.

8. **c**
   Factual recall
   Rationale: The terms in the question and listed as possible answers need to be defined to answer the question.

9. **b**
   Factual recall
   Rationale: The terms in the question and listed as possible answers need to be defined to answer the question. The question is a definition of tone.

10. **c**
    Application and concept identification
    Rationale: The question identifies the genetic tendency for fast twitch and slow twitch fiber types in muscles. The wrong answers are not logical in relation to the facts in the question or misuse terminology in relation to other terms in the sentence. This is a common strategy for creating wrong answers.

11. **a**
    Application and concept identification
    Rationale: Postural muscles are fatigue resistant and usually made of a higher percentage of slow twitch red fibers. To affect these muscles, a sustained force at threshold stimulus needs to be applied.

12. **b**
    Factual recall
    Rationale: The terms in the question and listed as possible answers need to be defined to answer the question. The structure of capillaries is long and winding to accommodate the changes in muscle shape.

13. **d**
    Factual recall
    Rationale: The connective tissue is continuous with muscle fibers. The three incorrect answers describe functions of muscles.

14. **a**
    Factual recall
    Rationale: The terms in the question and listed as possible answers need to be defined to answer the question.

15. **b**
    Application and concept identification
    Rationale: The question is asking for the rationale for the massage method described. Slow stretching affects the viscous aspect of the connective tissue more than the neurologic or chemical action of muscle fibers. Slow stretching has minimal effect on blood flow. Answer c is incorrect because slow stretching would increase, not decrease, water binding.

16. **c**
Clinical reasoning/synthesis
Rationale: The facts in the question describe two different healing outcomes to a similar injury. Client A has near normal function while client B has dysfunction. There needs to be a decision as to why this occurred based on correct information. The answers need to be analyzed in relation to the question and general factual data about tissue healing. Only answer c meets these criteria. Limiting exercise and wrapping the area would result in less mobility, and client A had near normal function. Satellite cell activity results in replacement during healing, not increased scar development. Increased circulation and decreased adhesions result in mobility, not rigidity.

17. **a**
Factual recall
Rationale: The terms in the question and listed as possible answers need to be defined to answer the question.

18. **d**
Application and concept identification
Rationale: The question is asking for an understanding of movement, muscle attachments, and terminology. All the terminology needs to be defined to understand the question and possible answers. The correct answer needs to be identified based on muscle anatomy and physiology. The wrong answers use all the right words in the wrong context. This is common strategy for writing wrong answers. Only answer d correctly describes the reason for the increased tenderness on palpation.

19. **b**
Factual recall
Rationale: The terms listed as possible answers need to be defined to answer the question. The question defines a function of pennate muscle shape.

20. **c**
Application and concept identification
Rationale: The question describes a myotatic unit. The answers listed are the components of myotatic units, and these terms need to be defined. The agonist for abduction requires that the antagonist (the adductor) relax to allow for the movement. If this is not happening, then the antagonist is the likely cause.

21. **a**
Factual recall
Rationale: The terms listed as possible answers need to be defined to answer the question. The question provides a definition of myotatic units.

22. **b**
Factual recall
Rationale: The terms listed as possible answers need to be defined to answer the question. The question provides a definition of the flexor reflex.

23. **b**
Application and concept identification
Rationale: The action described in the question stimulated the protective action of the tendon reflex. The question asks for a correlation of the reflex physiology to an actual situation. An understanding of agonist and antagonist interaction and the response patterns of all the reflexes listed in the possible answers is necessary to identify the correct answer.

24. **c**
Factual recall
Rationale: The terms listed as possible answers need to be defined to answer the question. The question provides a function of smooth muscle.

25. **d**
Factual recall
Rationale: This question is representative of hundreds of questions that can be written about muscle anatomy and physiology. To answer these types of questions there needs to be a factual basis about attachments, innervation, function, myotatic unit, common trigger points, and referred pain patterns of the individual muscles. This question asks for referred pain pattern.

26. **b**
Factual recall
Rationale: This question is representative of hundreds of questions that can be written about muscle anatomy and physiology. To answer these types of questions there needs to be a factual basis about attachments, innervation, function, myotatic unit, common trigger points, and referred pain patterns of the individual muscles. This question asks for function.

27. **a**
    Factual recall
    Rationale: This question is representative of hundreds of questions that can be written about muscle anatomy and physiology. To answer these types of questions there needs to be a factual basis about attachments, innervation, function, myotatic unit, common trigger points, and referred pain patterns of the individual muscles. This question asks for function of a group based on location.

28. **c**
    Factual recall
    Rationale: This question is representative of hundreds of questions that can be written about muscle anatomy and physiology. To answer these types of questions there needs to be a factual basis about attachments, innervation, function, myotatic unit, common trigger points, and referred pain patterns of the individual muscles. This question asks for referred pain pattern.

29. **b**
    Factual recall
    Rationale: This question is representative of hundreds of questions that can be written about muscle anatomy and physiology. To answer these types of questions there needs to be a factual basis about attachments, innervation, function, myotatic unit, common trigger points and referred pain patterns of the individual muscles. This question asks for myotatic unit interaction.

30. **d**
    Factual recall
    Rationale: This question is representative of hundreds of questions that can be written about muscle anatomy and physiology. To answer these types of questions there needs to be a factual basis about attachments, innervation, function, myotatic unit, common trigger points, and referred pain patterns of the individual muscles. This question asks for function.

31. **a**
    Factual recall
    Rationale: This question is representative of hundreds of questions that can be written about muscle anatomy and physiology. To answer these types of questions there needs to be a factual basis about attachments, innervation, function, myotatic unit, common trigger points, and referred pain patterns of the individual muscles. This question ask for referred pain pattern.

32. **c**
    Factual recall
    Rationale: This question is representative of hundreds of questions that can be written about muscle anatomy and physiology. To answer these types of questions there needs to be a factual basis about attachments, innervation, function, myotatic unit, common trigger points, and referred pain patterns of the individual muscles. This question asks for origin and insertion.

33. **a**
    Factual recall
    Rationale: This question is representative of hundreds of questions that can be written about muscle anatomy and physiology. To answer these types of questions there needs to be a factual basis about attachments, innervation, function, myotatic unit, common trigger points, and referred pain patterns of the individual muscles. This question asks about nerve supply.

34. **b**
    Factual recall
    Rationale: This question is representative of hundreds of questions that can be written about muscle anatomy and physiology. To answer these types of questions there needs to be a factual basis about attachments, innervation, function, myotatic unit, common trigger points, and referred pain patterns of the individual muscles. This question asks about function.

35. **c**
    Factual recall
    Rationale: This question is representative of hundreds of questions that can be written about muscle anatomy and physiology. To answer these types of questions there needs to be a factual basis about attachments, innervation, function, myotatic unit, common trigger points, and referred pain patterns of the individual muscles. This question asks about function.

36. **d**
    Factual recall
    Rationale: This question is representative of hundreds of questions that can be written about muscle anatomy and physiology. To answer these types of questions there needs to be a factual basis about attachments, innervation, function, myotatic unit, common trigger points, and referred pain patterns of the individual muscles. The question is asking for myotatic unit, particularly the antagonist to the subscapularis.

37. **c**
Factual recall
Rationale: This question is representative of hundreds of questions that can be written about muscle anatomy and physiology. To answer these types of questions there needs to be a factual basis about attachments, innervation, function, myotatic unit, common trigger points, and referred pain patterns of the individual muscles. This question is asking for impaired function of an antagonist pattern.

38. **d**
Factual recall
Rationale: This question is representative of hundreds of questions that can be written about muscle anatomy and physiology. To answer these types of questions there needs to be a factual basis about attachments, innervation, function, myotatic unit, common trigger points, and referred pain patterns of the individual muscles. This question describes a muscle location.

39. **c**
Factual recall
Rationale: This question is representative of hundreds of questions that can be written about muscle anatomy and physiology. To answer these types of questions there needs to be a factual basis about attachments, innervation, function, myotatic unit, common trigger points, and referred pain patterns of the individual muscles. This question asks for myotatic unit.

40. **a**
Clinical reasoning/synthesis
Rationale: The facts presented in the question are: extended contraction of the muscles used to grip (the flexor group of the forearm and the intrinsic muscles of the palm) and inhibition of the wrist extensors. The possible answers provide a reason for this condition. Each needs to be analyzed to determine the correct use of terminology and logical information based on the facts of the question.

41. **b**
Factual recall
Rationale: This question is representative of hundreds of questions that can be written about muscle anatomy and physiology. To answer these types of questions there needs to be a factual basis about attachments, innervation, function, myotatic unit, common trigger points, and referred pain patterns of the individual muscles. This question asks for location.

42. **c**
Factual recall
Rationale: This question is representative of hundreds of questions that can be written about muscle anatomy and physiology. To answer these types of questions there needs to be a factual basis about attachments, innervation, function, myotatic unit, common trigger points, and referred pain patterns of the individual muscles. This question describes function.

43. **d**
Factual recall
Rationale: This question is representative of hundreds of questions that can be written about muscle anatomy and physiology. To answer these types of questions there needs to be a factual basis about attachments, innervation, function, myotatic unit, common trigger points, and referred pain patterns of the individual muscles. This question asks for location.

44. **b**
Factual recall
Rationale: This question is representative of hundreds of questions that can be written about muscle anatomy and physiology. To answer these types of questions there needs to be a factual basis about attachments, innervation, function, myotatic unit, common trigger points, and referred pain patterns of the individual muscles. This question asks for function.

45. **a**
Factual recall
Rationale: This question is representative of hundreds of questions that can be written about muscle anatomy and physiology. To answer these types of questions there needs to be a factual basis about attachments, innervation, function, myotatic unit, common trigger points, and referred pain patterns of the individual muscles. This question asks for myotatic unit.

46. **c**
Factual recall
Rationale: This question is representative of hundreds of questions that can be written about muscle anatomy and physiology. To answer these types of questions there needs to be a factual basis about attachments, innervation, function, myotatic unit, common trigger points, and referred pain patterns of the individual muscles. This question asks for function.

47. **d**
    Factual recall
    Rationale: This question is representative of hundreds of questions that can be written about muscle anatomy and physiology. To answer these types of questions there needs to be a factual basis about attachments, innervation, function, myotatic unit, common trigger points, and referred pain patterns of the individual muscles. This question asks for myotatic unit.

48. **c**
    Factual recall
    Rationale: This question is representative of hundreds of questions that can be written about muscle anatomy and physiology. To answer these types of questions there needs to be a factual basis about attachments, innervation, function, myotatic unit, common trigger points, and referred pain patterns of the individual muscles. This question asks for function and location.

49. **a**
    Factual recall
    Rationale: This question is representative of hundreds of questions that can be written about muscle anatomy and physiology. To answer these types of questions there needs to be a factual basis about attachments, innervation, function, myotatic unit, common trigger points, and referred pain patterns of the individual muscles. This question asks for function.

50. **b**
    Factual recall
    Rationale: This question is representative of hundreds of questions that can be written about muscle anatomy and physiology. To answer these types of questions there needs to be a factual basis about attachments, innervation, function, myotatic unit, common trigger points, and referred pain patterns of the individual muscles. This question asks for function.

51. **d**
    Factual recall
    Rationale: This question is representative of hundreds of questions that can be written about muscle anatomy and physiology. To answer these types of questions there needs to be a factual basis about attachments, innervation, function, myotatic unit, common trigger points, and referred pain patterns of the individual muscles. This question asks for function.

52. **b**
    Factual recall
    Rationale: This question is representative of hundreds of questions that can be written about muscle anatomy and physiology. To answer these types of questions there needs to be a factual basis about attachments, innervation, function, myotatic unit, common trigger points, and referred pain patterns of the individual muscles. This question asks for myotatic unit.

53. **c**
    Factual recall
    Rationale: This question is representative of hundreds of questions that can be written about muscle anatomy and physiology. To answer these types of questions there needs to be a factual basis about attachments, innervation, function, myotatic unit, common trigger points, and referred pain patterns of the individual muscles. This question asks for location.

54. **b**
    Application and concept identification
    Rationale: The question is describing the pain-spasm-pain cycle.

55. **d**
    Factual recall
    Rationale: This question is representative of many questions that can be written about muscle pathology. To answer these types of questions there needs to be a factual basis about attachments, innervation, function, myotatic unit, common trigger points, and referred pain patterns of the individual muscles along with medications, common pathology, and methods of treatment. This question is asking for identification of antiinflammatory medication.

56. **a**
    Factual recall
    Rationale: This question is representative of the many questions that can be written about muscle pathology. To answer these types of questions there needs to be a factual basis about attachments, innervation, function, myotatic unit, common trigger points, and referred pain patterns of the individual muscles along with medications, common pathology, and methods of treatment. This question is asking for the cautions for applying massage. An analgesic is a painkiller.

57. **c**
Application and concept identification
Rationale: The question requires an understanding of the pathologies listed correlated with the benefits of a general massage. The three wrong answers present either contraindications or complex conditions requiring specific intervention. Muscle tension headache commonly responds well to general massage, which generates a parasympathetic effect.

58. **b**
Factual recall
Rationale: This question is representative of hundreds of questions that can be written about muscle pathology. This question is asking for the cautions for applying massage. The three wrong answers indicate general contraindications. Only myositis ossificans has a regional contraindication.

59. **d**
Clinical reasoning/synthesis
Rationale: The facts are related to the condition of fibromyalgia. The decision is what is the best massage approach to use. Fibromyalgia is muscle pain syndrome, which responds best to general massage to support sleep and relieve pain symptoms. Any type of massage that creates inflammation or excessively strains the system is contraindicated.

10

Biomechanics Basics

Questions

1. What type of contraction occurs when the muscle lengthens while under tension, changes in tension occur to control the descent of resistance, and joint angle increases?

   a. Isometric eccentric
   b. Isotonic concentric
   c. Isotonic concentric
   d. Isotonic eccentric

2. The amount of force on a specific area is called _____.

   a. Pressure
   b. Inertia
   c. Acceleration
   d. Center of gravity

3. A person who is maintaining an upright posture while reaching for an object is displaying _____.

   a. Static balance
   b. Dynamic balance
   c. Static equilibrium
   d. Inertia

4. Which of the following statements would describe the least amount of balance?

   a. Greater weight centered over a large base of support
   b. The center of gravity outside the base of support
   c. A low center of gravity with rotation around the axis
   d. An enlarged base of support in response to oncoming force

5. The most efficient movement of the body into forward motion begins with the _____.

   a. Legs
   b. Arms
   c. Head
   d. Hips

6. Which of the following would most often be considered the fulcrum?

   a. Quadriceps muscles
   b. Radius
   c. Deltoid ligament
   d. Glenohumeral joint

7. When one is carrying a massage table from the car to the office, what is the responsibility of the muscles?

   a. Create a lever to distribute the load
   b. Exert effort to move the load
   c. Provide a fulcrum for the lever
   d. Maintain static balance

8. Since the body movements of the limb most often require rapid movement and insertions of the muscles close to the joint, which lever type is most often found?

   a. First-class lever
   b. Second-class lever
   c. Third-class lever
   d. Combined lever

Answers are on pages 85–87.

9. *During normal gait in the adult, the lumbar rotation is countered by a cervical spine rotation in the opposite direction for what reason?*

   a. To keep the eyes on a level plane and the head oriented forward with the trunk

   b. To maintain the same-side counterbalance action of the arms and legs

   c. To coordinate the lever action of the elbows with the knees

   d. To activate the second-class lever system of the lift of the heel when moving onto the toes

10. *An individual was running up stairs carrying a heavy briefcase in the left hand. Later that day the person felt increased tension in the left biceps muscle. Two days later, during a regular massage session, the client describes weakness and heaviness in one leg when walking up stairs or a hill. If normal gait reflexes are functioning, where would assessment likely find an inhibited muscle pattern?*

    a. Right arm extensors

    b. Left hip flexors

    c. Right hip flexors

    d. Left hip extensors

11. *During normal gait, when one foot is in contact with the floor it is called the _____.*

    a. Stance phase

    b. Double stance

    c. Swing phase

    d. Double swing

12. *Which of the following aspects of the gait cycle would result in most concentric contraction of the plantar flexors?*

    a. Heel strike

    b. Mid-stance

    c. Toe-off preswing

    d. Mid-swing

13. *When one is correctly moving from a seated to a standing position, the head moves forward and the hips bend, which moves the torso forward, then _____.*

    a. The arms are contracted and push the body upright into a standing position

    b. The legs lift the body from the semisquat position into a standing position

    c. The leg muscles tense to provide stability while the back muscles straighten the torso

    d. The arms support the torso on the thighs so that the psoas and gluteal muscles can lift the body into a standing position

14. *After tripping down a stair, but not falling, a client describes a sudden onset of pain during twisting and reaching movements. Which type of biomechanical dysfunction is most likely to be occurring?*

    a. Neuromuscular

    b. Myofascial

    c. Joint related

    d. Capsular pattern

15. *A reversible limitation of range of movement that occurs as a result of change in connective tissue following long-term muscle spasms is called _____.*

    a. Nonoptimal motor function

    b. Capsular pattern

    c. Regional postural muscular imbalance

    d. Functional block

16. *A client reports information during the history-taking process, which is confirmed with physical assessment, indicating that postural muscles are moderately short with mild connective tissue changes. Antagonist muscle patterns show some inhibition. What degree of imbalance is being observed?*

    a. First degree

    b. Second degree

    c. Third degree

    d. Fourth degree

17. *A client has been referred by the physician for massage. The diagnosis is functional stress with second-degree distortion of motor function. Which of the following symptoms would the client likely be experiencing?*

    a. Minor recruitment of synergist muscles but not postural change
    b. Weakness of antagonist patterns and specific nonoptimal movement
    c. Fatigue with daily activities, mild pain, and localized functional blocks
    d. Instability of vertebral motion segments with painful muscle tension and connective tissue shortening

18. *A client experienced an auto accident 4 years ago that resulted in a bulging disk at L-4. The injury has since healed with minimal difficulties. During assessment, palpation indicates a moderate decrease in pliability of the lumbar dorsal fascia and mild shortening in the lumbar muscles. Forward flexion and rotation of the lumbar area are mildly impaired. Massage was focused to reduce the muscle shortening in the lumbar area and increase connective tissue pliability. Immediately after the massage the client reported increased mobility but within 15 minutes began to complain of lower back pain. What is the most likely explanation for this occurrence?*

    a. A shift of the condition from second-degree functional stress to first-degree functional tension
    b. Increase in stability around the past injury
    c. Decrease in mobility in the area around the past injury
    d. Destabilization of resourceful compensation in lumbar area around past injury

19. *When a joint is moved so that the joint angle is decreased, what is occurring?*

    a. Prime movers and synergist concentrically contract. The antagonist eccentrically contracts while lengthening to allow the movement
    b. Prime movers concentrically contract with the antagonist so that synergists lengthen to allow movement
    c. Movement occurs as the antagonist contracts and prime movers eccentrically control the movement
    d. Resistance is applied to the fixators, providing the movement activating the prime movers

20. *A massage professional positions the client's body to assess the strength of the hip flexors. Which is the correct position for the hand applying resistance?*

    a. Near the hip
    b. At the ankle
    c. At the distal end of the femur
    d. On the tibia

21. *During joint movement and muscle strength assessment, it is important to isolate the movement to the jointed area being assessed. This is called _____.*

    a. Force
    b. Resistance
    c. Balance
    d. Stabilization

22. *Wrist flexion has a normal range of 0 to 80 degrees. A client is assessed with a range of motion of 100 degrees. This jointed area would be considered _____.*

    a. Balanced
    b. Hypermobile
    c. Hypomobile
    d. Inhibited

Answers are on pages 85–87.

23. *A client complains of joint pain in the knee and assessment indicates hypermobility with pain on passive movement. Which of the following would be the most appropriate treatment plan?*

    a. General massage to the body with specific muscle energy work and lengthening of the extensors and flexors of the knee
    b. General massage with regional contraindications to the knee area and referral for more appropriate diagnosis of possible capsular dysfunction
    c. Referral for diagnosis prior to any massage
    d. General massage with attention to friction methods at the joint capsule

24. *A client is experiencing an upper chest breathing pattern. Which of the following muscle(s) may test as short and too strong from this type of breathing?*

    a. Diaphragm
    b. Suprahyoids
    c. Scalenes
    d. Infraspinalis

25. *The typical range of motion in extension for the lumbar spine is _____.*

    a. 25 degrees
    b. 5 degrees
    c. 40 degrees
    d. 60 degrees

26. *A client complains of pain and tension in the lower back more to the left side. Physical assessment indicates that the pelvis is elevated on the left as compared to the right. The client also indicates difficulty raising the left arm over the head. Which of the following muscles may be involved?*

    a. Psoas
    b. Rectus abdominis
    c. Latissimus dorsi
    d. Semispinalis

27. *A client is having difficulty moving the head into cervical extension beyond 10 degrees. Which of the following cervical flexor muscles may be restricting mobility?*

    a. Longissimus capitis
    b. Sternocleidomastoid
    c. Splenius capitis
    d. Iliocostalis cervicis

28. *A client is unable to rotate the cervical area to turn the head past 20 degrees to the left. Muscle testing should indicate what?*

    a. Even strength on both sides
    b. Increased tension in the right cervical rotators
    c. Weakness in the right cervical rotators
    d. Increased strength in the cervical flexors

29. *Which of the following muscles is able to indirectly affect the sternoclavicular joint?*

    a. Deltoid
    b. Triceps
    c. Pectoralis minor
    d. Pectoralis major

30. *If the scapula remains fixed and immobile, what would result at the glenohumeral joint?*

    a. Range of motion would be limited
    b. Internal and external rotation would be enhanced
    c. Flexion would be unaffected
    d. Horizontal abduction would be the only limitation

31. *The glenohumeral joint is a good example to describe which of the following correct biomechanical principles?*

    a. When mobility increases, stability also increases
    b. When stability is less, mobility also decreases
    c. The more mobility, the less stability
    d. Mobility is supported before stability

32. *The primary function of the shoulder girdle muscles that have attachments at the axial skeleton, the scapula, and the clavicle is _____ .*

    a. Extension of the shoulder joint
    b. Stability of the scapula
    c. Mobility of the humerus
    d. Mobility of the glenohumeral joint

33. *A client is experiencing pain with any activity involving external or lateral rotation of the right shoulder. Range of motion is limited to 40 degrees. This condition has been coming on gradually. Muscle testing indicates weakness when resistance is applied to move the shoulder from external rotation to internal rotation. There is shortening in the muscles of internal rotation. Which of the following would be the most logical treatment plan?*

    a. Muscle energy methods to support lengthening of the infraspinatus and methods to increase tone in the subscapularis
    b. Deep massage to the rhomboids and stretching of the lumbar fascia
    c. Traction of the scapulothoracic junction
    d. Massage to reduce tension in the pectoralis major and latissimus dorsi with tapotement to increase tone in the infraspinatus and teres major

34. *A client has elbow flexion of 90 degrees. This is considered _____ .*

    a. Normal
    b. Hypermobility
    c. Hypomobility
    d. Instability

35. *A client is unable to turn the palm up past 45 degrees. Which of the following movements is hypomobile?*

    a. Supination
    b. Pronation
    c. Flexion
    d. Extension

36. *How is the area positioned and where is resistance applied to perform a muscle test for the normal function of the wrist flexors?*

    a. The elbow is flexed, and resistance is applied against the forearm
    b. The wrist is flexed, and resistance is applied against the palm of the hand
    c. The wrist is extended, and resistance is applied against the palm of the hand
    d. The wrist is flexed, and resistance is applied against the dorsal side of the hand

37. *When the left hip moves into flexion, what is the biomechanically correct movement of the pelvic girdle and the lumbar spine?*

    a. Anterior rotation for pelvic girdle and extension for lumbar spine
    b. Posterior rotation for pelvic girdle and flexion for lumbar spine
    c. Left lateral rotation for pelvic girdle and right lateral flexion for lumbar spine
    d. Left transverse rotation for pelvic girdle and external rotation of lumbar spine

38. *Concentric contraction occurs in which muscles when the thigh is flexed toward the trunk?*

    a. Hamstrings
    b. Gluteus maximus
    c. Iliopsoas
    d. Vastus lateralis

39. *A client lying prone is unable to lift the thigh off the table when attempting hip extension. Which muscle is not able to contract effectively?*

    a. Sartorius
    b. Adductor magnus
    c. Rectus femoris
    d. Semimembranosus

Answers are on pages 85–87.

40. A client is lying supine and observation indicates that the left leg is internally rotated. What should muscle testing reveal?

    a. Muscles that externally rotate the hip are short, and muscles that internally rotate the hip are inhibited
    b. Muscles that externally rotate the hip are inhibited, and muscles that internally rotate the hip are overly strong
    c. Gluteus medius should test weak
    d. Adductor longus should test weak

41. A massage practitioner wishes to assess the ability of the knee to move into slight internal and external rotation. How should the knee be positioned?

    a. Full extension
    b. 5 degrees of hyperextension
    c. 30 degrees of flexion
    d. 10 degrees of flexion

42. The knee is placed in 100 degrees of extension and the client is asked to hold this position. Resistance is applied to the concentrically contracting muscles. Pain and weakness are felt. What is a logical explanation for this?

    a. The hamstring muscle group is weak
    b. The Q angle is being altered in a lateral direction by the contraction of the vastus medialis
    c. The popliteus muscle has been unable to unlock the screw-home mechanism
    d. The quadriceps muscle group is unable to effectively hold a contraction against resistance

43. A client experienced a second-degree ankle sprain when the foot was forced into inversion. Which of the following muscles would have experienced an extension injury?

    a. Peroneus longus
    b. Soleus
    c. Flexor digitorum longus
    d. Interossei

Answers and Discussion

1. **d**
   Factual recall
   Rationale: As in all questions, the terminology needs to be defined to correctly interpret the question and possible answers. The question is the definition of an isotonic eccentric contraction.

2. **a**
   Factual recall
   Rationale: After one defines the possible answers, the question is recognized as a definition of pressure.

3. **b**
   Factual recall
   Rationale: After one defines the possible answers, the question describes dynamic balance.

4. **b**
   Factual recall
   Rationale: After one analyzes the possible answers in relation to balance principles and compares them to the question, which asks for a condition that increases instability, only answer b is logical.

5. **c**
   Factual recall
   Rationale: The weight of the head carries the body forward.

6. **d**
   Application and concept identification
   Rationale: A fulcrum is a fixed point around which a lever rotates. Only the joint can be a fulcrum; bones are levers and muscles provide force.

7. **b**
   Application and concept identification
   Rationale: The question describes an action and asks for muscle function. Muscles exert a force to generate effort to overcome resistance.

8. **c**
   Factual recall
   Rationale: The lever types need to be defined. There is no combined lever type. A third-class lever provides the greatest speed.

9. **a**
   Application and concept identification
   Rationale: Visual input during gait require that the eyes remain forward and be kept level.

10. **b**
    Clinical reasoning/synthesis
    Rationale: The question requires an analysis of normal gait patterns against the disrupted gait described in the question. The arms counterbalance the legs, with the right arm counterbalancing the left leg and vice versa. This would mean that when the shoulder flexors contract on the right, the thigh flexors on the left are also contracting. If the tension in the biceps muscle on the left has increased, it would inhibit the thigh flexors on the left and the thigh flexors on the right would increase in tone.

11. **a**
    Factual recall
    Rationale: The entire gait cycle needs to be understood to answer the question. The answers name certain aspects of gait. When the foot is on the floor it is the stance phase. There is no double swing during gait.

12. **c**
    Factual recall
    Rationale: This question requires interpretation of the terminology and understanding of muscle involvement creating the steps in the gait cycle listed as answers. Plantar flexors move the foot onto the toes, therefore toe-off preswing is the correct answer.

13. **b**
    Factual recall.
    Rationale: The question is asking for the sequential steps in moving from a seated to a standing position.

14. **a**
    Application and concept identification
    Rationale: To answer the question, one needs to define the four types of dysfunction, then relate to the facts presented. Because of the recent onset in response to a slight trauma, answer a is the most logical.

15. **d**
Factual recall
Rationale: The question is the definition of functional block.

16. **b**
Factual recall
Rationale: The question is describing a second-degree pattern.

17. **c**
Factual recall
Rationale: The question is asking for symptoms related to the diagnosis.

18. **d**
Clinical reasoning/synthesis
Rationale: The case study provides history, assessment data, methods used, and outcomes. The answers need to be analyzed in relation to the facts in the question. Since the condition changed from reduced range of motion without pain to increased range of motion but onset of pain, a shift from a second-degree to a first-degree dysfunction would not be logical. With mobility increasing, stability would decrease around the area. Answer d describes a change in compensation patterns and is the most logical reason for the pain.

19. **a**
Factual recall
Rationale: All the terms need to be defined and the question and the possible answer interpreted. This question is an example of terminology usage. The wrong answers are misusing the language.

20. **c**
Application and concept identification
Rationale: This question is representative of many different questions that can be written about biomechanical assessment and intervention. Resistance is applied to the distal end of the lever.

21. **d**
Factual recall
Rationale: The question defines stabilization.

22. **b**
Factual recall
Rationale: Range of motion beyond normal is considered hypermobile.

23. **b**
Clinical reasoning/synthesis
Rationale: Facts presented in the question are: knee joint pain with hypermobility and pain with passive movement. Facts provided by the textbook include: the knee is moving beyond 150 degrees of flexion and 135 degrees of extension. Pain on passive movement is often a joint dysfunction or nerve entrapment. The question asks for the best massage intervention based on this condition. The outcome is assumed to be a reversal of the condition. Answer a would increase the hypermobility. Answer b provides massage but refers the client for specific work on the knee since joint or nerve involvement is indicated by the assessment. This is the best answer. Answer c is too conservative, and answer d is too aggressive.

24. **c**
Application and concept identification
Rationale: The question is asking for a condition of a muscle group in response to a repetitive strain to the scalenes caused by the inappropriate breathing pattern.

25. **a**
Factual recall
Rationale: This question is representative of the many questions that can be written about range of motion. The degrees of movement for each joint need to be remembered to answer this type of question.

26. **c**
Application and concept identification
Rationale: The question asks for muscle involvement based on symptoms and assessment. To answer this type of question it is necessary to understand muscle anatomy and physiology along with myotatic units presented in Chapter 9. Then the muscle information needs to be integrated into biomechanical function. The information from the question indicates the latissimus dorsi.

27. **b**
Factual recall
Rationale: This question is representative of the many questions that can be written about range of motion. The degrees of movement for each joint and the muscles that produce the movement identified need to be remembered to answer this type of question. In this question only sternocleidomastoid is a cervical flexor.

28. **b**
Factual recall
Rationale: This question is representative of the many questions that can be written about range of motion. The degrees of movement for each joint and the muscles that produce the movement identified need to be remembered to answer this type of question. In this question restricted mobility on the left should indicate shortened and contracted muscles on the right.

29. **d**
Factual recall
Rationale: This question requires knowledge of the particular joint and the muscle that is either directly or indirectly working on the joint. Information about all the muscles listed as possible answers is necessary to eliminate wrong answers. Only the pectoralis major exerts influence on the sternoclavicular joint.

30. **a**
Application and concept identification
Rationale: The entire shoulder complex moves as a unit.

31. **c**
Application and concept identification
Rationale: A joint function is provided to identify a biomechanical principle. Information about the glenohumeral joint design is necessary to answer the question. Since this joint is one with the most mobility, answer c is the most logical.

32. **b**
Factual recall
Rationale: The question is asking for the function of a group of muscles in terms of biomechanics.

33. **d**
Clinical reasoning/synthesis
Rationale: The facts presented by the question are: right shoulder pain on external rotation with a slow onset. Range of motion is 40 degrees and normal is 90 degrees. Infraspinatus, posterior deltoid, and teres minor are inhibited by the subscapularis, pectoralis major, latissimus dorsi, teres major, and anterior deltoid. The correct answer would need to bring a reversal of the condition in a safe and conservative manner. Each answer has to have the terminology interpreted. Only answer d addresses the muscle listed as causal and applies proper methods to normalize the condition.

34. **c**
Factual recall
Rationale: Normal elbow flexion is 150 degrees, so the joint is hypomobile.

35. **a**
Application and concept identification
Rationale: The action limited is supination.

36. **b**
Factual recall
Rationale: This question is representative of proper positioning to isolate and test muscles.

37. **a**
Factual recall
Rationale: The hip, pelvic girdle, and lumbar spine are in a closed kinematic chain.

38. **c**
Factual recall
Rationale: The question describes a function of the iliopsoas.

39. **d**
Factual recall
Rationale: The question asks for what muscle is testing weak for hip extension. Semimembranosus is the only listed muscle involved in hip extension.

40. **b**
Application and concept identification
Rationale: The question is asking for a relationship between observed internal rotation and the outcome of muscle testing. Answer a reverses the information. The two muscles in answers c and d are not involved in the movement described.

41. **c**
Factual recall
Rationale: The loose packed position of the knee is at about 30 degrees of flexion, allowing for the movement of internal and external rotation.

42. **d**
Application and concept identification
Rationale: The concentrically contracting group of muscles in the knee being held in extension is the quadriceps.

43. **a**
Application and concept identification
Rationale: The peroneus longus is the only muscle that would be overstretched by this action.

11

Integumentary, Cardiovascular, Lymphatic, and Immune Systems

Questions

1. *Which of the following functions of the integumentary system is supported by maintaining sanitary procedures?*

   a. Protecting against water loss
   b. Detecting sensory stimuli
   c. Preventing entry of bacteria and viruses
   d. Excreting sweat and salts

2. *The outer layer of the skin is called the _____.*

   a. Epidermis
   b. Dermis
   c. Superficial fascia
   d. Keratin

3. *The pigment of our skin is produced by _____.*

   a. Dermis
   b. Stratum corneum
   c. Adipose
   d. Melanocytes

4. *Erector pili muscles are attached to _____.*

   a. Nails
   b. Hair
   c. Fat cells
   d. Lunula

5. *Sebum is produced by _____.*

   a. Sweat glands
   b. Mammary glands
   c. Sebaceous glands
   d. Root plexus

6. *Sweat produced by which of the following glands has the strongest odor?*

   a. Eccrine
   b. Apocrine
   c. Ceruminous
   d. Sebaceous

7. *A massage practitioner notices that a client's skin has a yellowish gold color. This would be an indication of _____.*

   a. Cyanosis
   b. Anemia
   c. Fever
   d. Jaundice

8. *Which of the following is a contagious skin disease?*

   a. Impetigo
   b. Alopecia
   c. Scleroderma
   d. Vitiligo

Answers are on pages 93–95.

9. Which of the following benign skin growths has the most potential for becoming malignant?

   a. Angioma
   b. Mole
   c. Lipoma
   d. Seborrheic keratosis

10. A massage professional identifies a few small lumps in the axillary area of a female client. What might be a pathologic concern?

    a. Basal cell carcinoma
    b. Candidiasis
    c. Psoriasis
    d. Fibrocystic disease

11. The heart muscle is called the _____.

    a. Pericardium
    b. Myocardium
    c. Epicardium
    d. Endocardium

12. Which of the following heart valves controls the flow of blood from the ventricles into the aorta?

    a. Atrioventricular
    b. Mitral
    c. Tricuspid
    d. Semilunar

13. Which of the following vessels carries blood to the lungs?

    a. Aorta
    b. Superior vena cava
    c. Pulmonary trunk
    d. Inferior vena cava

14. A client has a history of heart attack and has reduced blood flow to the heart. Which of the following vessels is most involved?

    a. Coronary
    b. Left external carotid
    c. Celiac
    d. Renal

15. What is the first heart chamber to receive blood from the superior and inferior venae cavae?

    a. Right ventricle
    b. Right atrium
    c. Left ventricle
    d. Left atrium

16. Which portion of the cardiac cycle performs relaxation of the ventricles during filling?

    a. Sinoatrial node
    b. Systole
    c. AV bundle
    d. Diastole

17. A client complains of pooling of blood in the lower extremities. Which of the following circumstances would be a likely cause?

    a. Increased walking
    b. Lying with the feet above the heart
    c. Standing still for extended periods
    d. Regular deep breathing

18. During a general massage the massage practitioner notices that the dorsalis pedis pulse is weaker on the left. Where is the practitioner palpating?

    a. Upper arm
    b. Wrist
    c. Knee
    d. Ankle

19. Which of the following would be an indication for referral?

    a. A radial pulse of 85 beats per minute
    b. A femoral pulse of 55 beats per minute
    c. A carotid pulse of 70 beats per minute
    d. A dorsalis pedis pulse of 52 beats per minute

20. A client reports commonly having a blood pressure of 90/50. What would this condition be called?

    a. Tachycardia
    b. Hypertension
    c. Hypotension
    d. Bradycardia

21. *After a 1-hour massage focused on relaxation, a client becomes dizzy when sitting up. What is the likely cause?*

    a. Stimulation of baroreceptors
    b. Increase of sympathetic stimulation
    c. Pulse rate of 65 beats per minute
    d. Decrease in parasympathetic tone

22. *Applying deep pressure during massage to the neck near the sternocleidomastoid muscles could compress which artery?*

    a. Basilar
    b. External carotid
    c. Axillary
    d. Mesenteric

23. *Deep extended pressure behind the knee is contraindicated because of potential damage to which artery?*

    a. Celiac
    b. Femoral
    c. Popliteal
    d. Posterior tibial

24. *Which of the following veins is located in the arm?*

    a. Basilic
    b. Jugular
    c. Renal
    d. Iliac

25. *A client has had surgery for varicose veins in the legs. Which vein was removed?*

    a. Azygous
    b. Brachiocephalic
    c. Hepatic
    d. Saphenous

26. *Which of the following contributes to hematopoiesis?*

    a. Erythrocyte
    b. Monocyte
    c. Stem cell
    d. Thrombocyte

27. *Which of the following is a temporary deficiency or diminished supply of blood to a tissue?*

    a. Aneurysm
    b. Embolus
    c. Blockage of a vessel
    d. Ischemia

28. *A pulmonary embolism may begin as _____.*

    a. Deep vein thrombosis
    b. Hemophilia
    c. Angina pectoris
    d. Arrhythmia

29. *Clear interstitial tissue fluid is called _____.*

    a. Lymphocytes
    b. Lymph
    c. Plasma
    d. Fibrin

30. *Both lymphatic ducts empty lymph fluid into the _____.*

    a. Mediastinal nodes
    b. Subclavian veins
    c. Mesenteric artery
    d. Cisterna chyli

31. *Massage that provides a pumping compression to the foot encourages lymphatic flow because _____.*

    a. The palmar plexus is stimulated
    b. The parotid nodes are drained
    c. The plantar plexus is stimulated
    d. The mammary plexus is stimulated

32. *Which of the following acts to store lymphocytes and blood?*

    a. Thymus
    b. Peyer's patches
    c. Bone marrow
    d. Spleen

Answers are on pages 93–95.

33. *Which of the following is considered contagious?*

    a. Hodgkin's disease
    b. Mononucleosis
    c. Leukemia
    d. Lymphoma

34. *A person had the measles as a child and is no longer susceptible. This is called _____.*

    a. Nonspecific immunity
    b. Immune deficiency
    c. Specific immunity
    d. Phagocytosis

35. *Antigens are destroyed or suppressed by _____.*

    a. The thymus
    b. Antibodies
    c. Nonspecific immunity
    d. Lymph nodes

36. *The immune function of mucus results because _____.*

    a. It is sticky
    b. It creates inflammation
    c. Of phagocytosis
    d. It washes pathogens from the body

37. *Allergy is a condition of _____.*

    a. Immune system suppression
    b. Lack of T-cell activity
    c. Overactive immune response
    d. Immune deficiency

38. *A client has been experiencing ongoing work and family stress and cannot seem to recover from an upper respiratory infection. What is the most logical cause?*

    a. Ongoing stress increases natural killer cells
    b. Ongoing stress supports the development of autoimmune disease
    c. Ongoing stress suppresses T-cell activity
    d. Decrease in cortisol suppresses the immune system

39. *What is the contribution of the urinary system to immune function?*

    a. Protective acid balance
    b. Mechanical barrier
    c. Development of lymphocytes
    d. Nutrient delivery to cells

40. *Which of the following is considered sterilization for aseptic pathogen control?*

    a. Iodine
    b. Chlorine
    c. Alcohol
    d. Extreme heat

41. *The most likely transmission route for both HIV and hepatitis is _____.*

    a. Handshaking
    b. Body fluids
    c. Environmental contact
    d. Droplets in the air

42. *A client is immune suppressed. The physician has provided approval for massage. What would be the best massage treatment plan?*

    a. General massage with specific use of stimulation techniques to encourage sympathetic dominance
    b. General massage with a focus on aggressive lymphatic drainage
    c. General massage with active stretching to encourage parasympathetic dominance
    d. General massage to support nonspecific homeostatic regulation and restorative sleep

Answers and Discussion

1. **c**
   Application and concept identification
   Rationale: Sanitary practices support the protective barrier of the skin.

2. **a**
   Factual recall
   Rationale: The terms need to be defined to identify the correct answer. When this is done epidermis is identified as the outer layer of the skin.

3. **d**
   Factual recall
   Rationale: The terms need to be defined to identify the correct answer.

4. **b**
   Factual recall
   Rationale: The location of the erector pili muscles is at the hair root.

5. **c**
   Factual recall
   Rationale: The terms all need to be defined to answer the question.

6. **b**
   Factual recall
   Rationale: The terms need to be defined and the different types of sweat understood to answer the question.

7. **d**
   Application and concept identification
   Rationale: Color changes in the skin can be an indication of pathology. A yellow cast may indicate jaundice.

8. **a**
   Factual recall
   Rationale: It is important to be able to recognize the various skin pathologies. Contagious skin diseases are especially important to recognize. All of the listed skin pathologies should be defined, then impetigo emerges as the correct answer.

9. **b**
   Factual recall
   Rationale: It is important to be able to recognize the various skin pathologies. Those with the potential to malignant skin diseases are especially important to recognize. All of the listed skin pathologies should be defined, then a mole emerges as the correct answer.

10. **d**
    Factual recall
    Rationale: It is important to be able to recognize the various integumentary pathologies. All of the listed pathologies should be defined, then fibrocystic disease emerges as the correct answer.

11. **b**
    Factual recall
    Rationale: The terms need to be defined to identify the correct answer.

12. **d**
    Factual recall
    Rationale: The question provides information to differentiate among the heart valves listed as possible answers.

13. **c**
    Factual recall
    Rationale: The location and function of all the vessels listed as possible answers need to be determined to answer the question.

14. **a**
    Application and concept identification
    Rationale: The question provides information about the location of the vessels by stating that the client had a heart attack and reduced blood flow to the heart. It is the coronary arteries that supply blood to the heart.

15. **b**
    Factual recall
    Rationale: Answering the question requires knowledge of blood flow through the heart.

16. **d**
    Factual recall
    Rationale: Answering the question requires knowledge about the cardiac cycle and the structures and/or functions listed as possible answers. Systole and diastole are part of the cardiac cycle, with diastole being the portion when the ventricles relax.

17. **c**
    Application and concept identification
    Rationale: The client has a reduced return of blood in the veins, and the correct answer explains why. The three wrong answers would increase blood flow in the veins. Only standing still for long periods would reduce blood flow.

18. **d**
Factual recall
Rationale: The question is representative of the many types of questions that can be developed about the arteries. This question asks for the location of a particular pulse point.

19. **a**
Application and concept identification
Rationale: A normal pulse is between 50 and 70 beats per minute. While 85 beats per minute is below what is considered tachycardia, it is faster than what is usually normal.

20. **c**
Factual recall
Rationale: A normal blood pressure is some-where around 120/80. The blood pressure described in the question is low, indicating hypotension.

21. **a**
Application and concept identification
Rationale: Care needs to be taken so that clients do not have low blood pressure after a massage. The three wrong answers would indicate an increase in blood pressure, and pressure on the baroreceptors can lower it.

22. **b**
Factual recall
Rationale: The question asks for the name of the artery located in the neck near a particular muscle that would interfere with blood flow. The arteries named in the wrong answers are not located in the neck.

23. **c**
Factual recall
Rationale: The question asks for the name of the artery located in the knee that is susceptible to compressive force. The arteries named in the wrong answers are not located behind the knee.

24. **a**
Factual recall
Rationale: The question is representative of many questions that can be developed about the location of blood vessels. This question asks for the identification of the basilic vein.

25. **d**
Factual recall
Rationale: The question is representative of many questions that can be developed about the location of blood vessels and pathology connected to them. This question asks for the identification of the saphenous vein.

26. **c**
Factual recall
Rationale: All the terms need to be defined to answer the question. Stem cells are involved in blood cell development.

27. **d**
Factual recall
Rationale: As in all of these types of questions, the terms have to be defined to answer the question.

28. **a**
Factual recall
Rationale: This question relates to pathology of the cardiovascular system. All the terms need to be defined to identify the correct answer and eliminate incorrect answers. In this question an embolism often begins as a thrombus

29. **b**
Factual recall
Rationale: As in all of these types of questions, the terms have to be defined to answer the question.

30. **b**
Factual recall
Rationale: As in all of these types of questions, the terms have to be defined to answer the question. Knowledge about the anatomy of the lymphatic system and the path of lymph flow is also required.

31. **c**
Application and concept identification
Rationale: An understanding is needed of the lymphatic plexus on the bottom of the foot and that compression to the area results in stimu-lation of lymphatic fluid movement.

32. **d**
Factual recall
Rationale: The question describes a function of the spleen.

33. **b**
Factual recall
Rationale: The question is asking about pathology of the lymphatic system. All of the diseases listed need to be defined and the one that is contagious identified.

34. **c**
Factual recall
Rationale: The question is an example of specific immunity.

35. **b**
Factual recall
Rationale: The question describes a function of antibodies.

36. **a**
Factual recall
Rationale: The correct answer describes the nonspecific immune defense of mucus.

37. **c**
Factual recall
Rationale: The correct answer is a definition of allergy.

38. **c**
Application and concept identification
Rationale: The question is asking for a correlation with immune suppression and stress levels. Only answer c is correct since stress tends to suppress the entire immune function through an increase in cortisol levels.

39. **a**
Factual recall
Rationale: This function of the urinary system acts to support nonspecific immunity.

40. **d**
Factual recall
Rationale: Sanitary measures support the immune system by isolating and destroying pathogens. Extreme heat kills most pathogens.

41. **b**
Factual recall
Rationale: These two diseases are transmitted in body fluids.

42. **d**
Clinical reasoning/synthesis
Rationale: The facts in the question indicate that the immune system is unable to fight pathogens. Precautions need to be taken to protect the client. No methods should be used to increase the stress response or strain the adaptive capacity of the client. Only the last answer meets these criteria.

CHAPTER

12

Respiratory, Digestive, Urinary, and Reproductive Systems

Questions

1. Which of the following is a mechanical action of inhalation and exhalation that draws oxygen into the lungs and releases carbon dioxide into the atmosphere?

   a. Breathing
   b. External respiration
   c. Internal respiration
   d. Egestion

2. The nasal cavity is separated into a right and left portion by _____.

   a. Nares
   b. Sinuses
   c. Ethmoid
   d. Septum

3. A client complains of both a congested nose and low back stiffness. What is the logical connection between the two?

   a. The respiratory mucus is too thin and allows bacteria to enter the body, causing a kidney infection
   b. The swell bodies in the nose are not able to function properly, so the normal movement during sleep is disrupted
   c. The olfactory nerves are increasing parasympathetic arousal, causing an increase in muscle tension
   d. Nasal congestion is blocking the sinus cavities and inner ear, changing muscle tone in the lower extremities

4. The air sacs in the lungs are called _____.

   a. Epiglottis
   b. Bronchioles
   c. Lobes
   d. Alveoli

5. A client is displaying behavior consistent with sympathetic autonomic nervous system dominance. What would be the state of the bronchioles?

   a. Bronchodilation
   b. Bronchoconstriction
   c. Pneumothorax
   d. Hyperventilation

6. Why would a person with a spinal cord injury at C-6 be able to breathe without a ventilator?

   a. The intercostal nerves exit at C-5
   b. The phrenic nerve originates at C-3
   c. The mediastinum is intact
   d. The pleural cavity is innervated at C-1

7. The external intercostal muscles create a vacuum in the thorax in which way?

   a. The upper ribs expand
   b. The ribs are pulled together
   c. The lower ribs are lifted up and out
   d. The diaphragm muscle arches upward

8. *During assessment a client is observed with mild tachypnea, tension in the muscles of the neck and shoulder, and nervousness. Which of the following is most true?*

   a. Nitrogen levels have risen and oxygen levels have decreased, creating a decrease in tidal volume

   b. Oxyhemoglobin is saturated with carbon dioxide and the muscles display tetany

   c. An increase in carbon dioxide in the blood is triggering sympathetic activation

   d. Oxygen levels have increased and carbon dioxide levels have dropped, predisposing to hyperventilation syndrome

9. *A client with a diagnosis of asthma is referred for massage. What would be the most likely benefits of massage?*

   a. Activation of the sympathetic nervous system would support bronchoconstriction

   b. Reduction in anxiety and increased mobility of the ribs

   c. Stimulation of the client's ability to inhale but inhibition of excessive exhalation

   d. Increase in tone of respiratory muscles, supporting effective exhalation

10. *Which of the following is contagious?*

    a. Tuberculosis

    b. Hayfever

    c. Emphysema

    d. Cystic fibrosis

11. *Massage methods that modulate the breathing rhythm also _____.*

    a. Predispose a person to pulmonary embolism

    b. Interfere with treatment for sleep apnea

    c. Interact with the autonomic nervous system

    d. Interfere with most meditation methods

12. *What supports addictive behavior related to food consumption?*

    a. Need for nutrients

    b. Pleasure sensations

    c. Energy requirement

    d. Peristalsis activation

13. *The abdominal cavity is lined with a mucous membrane called the _____.*

    a. Peritoneum

    b. Gastrointestinal tract

    c. Omentum

    d. Mesentery

14. *The enzyme amylase found in saliva is part of the digestion process for _____.*

    a. Proteins

    b. Fats

    c. Lipids

    d. Carbohydrates

15. *The folds in the stomach that expand when food is ingested are called _____.*

    a. Bolus

    b. Rugae

    c. Chyme

    d. Pylorus

16. *Which portion of the small intestine contains ducts from the liver, gallbladder, and pancreas?*

    a. Ileum

    b. Jejunum

    c. Duodenum

    d. Mesentery

17. *Which of the following acts as a digestive organ and also detoxifies the blood?*

    a. Pancreas

    b. Stomach

    c. Liver

    d. Gallbladder

18. *A major function of the large intestine is to _____.*

    a. Absorb water

    b. Concentrate bile

    c. Remove and store glycogen

    d. Convert amino acids

19. *Which of the following structures of the colon also contains lymphatic tissue?*

    a. Cecum
    b. Appendix
    c. Ascending colon
    d. Sigmoid colon

20. *A regular client reports various digestive upsets including dry mouth and constipation. The physician who wants a treatment plan and justification has cleared the client for massage. Which of the following would be the best plan to submit to the physician?*

    a. Stimulating massage coupled with teaching self-help breathing supporting an increase in oxygen and a decrease in carbon dioxide to support ongoing ANS sympathetic dominance
    b. General massage combined with deep massage to the colon to suppress peristalsis and break down concentrated fecal matter
    c. General massage focused to generate relaxation with diaphragmatic breathing and rhythmic stroking to the colon to stimulate peristalsis
    d. General massage to create parasympathetic dominance and lymphatic drainage, with visceral massage to the liver to increase detoxification and support upper chest breathing

21. *The food source that breaks down into amino acids is _____.*

    a. Protein
    b. Carbohydrate
    c. Fat
    d. Vitamins

22. *A client has severely limited all dietary fat. Which of the following might occur?*

    a. Inability to digest protein
    b. Difficulty with hormone production
    c. Interference with the absorption of water-soluble vitamins
    d. Decreased conversion of galactose

23. *Which of the following pathologies of the digestive system affects the liver?*

    a. Cystic fibrosis
    b. Diverticular disease
    c. Cirrhosis
    d. Gastritis

24. *Of the following, which is contagious?*

    a. Appendicitis
    b. Hepatitis
    c. Reflux esophagitis
    d. Irritable bowel syndrome

25. *Which of the following pathologic conditions is considered a medical emergency and requires immediate referral?*

    a. Gastroenteritis
    b. Peptic ulcer disease
    c. Inflammatory bowel disease
    d. Strangulated hernia

26. *Appropriate massage for the colon _____.*

    a. Begins at the ascending colon, ends at the rectum, and moves toward the cecum
    b. Begins at the sigmoid colon and ends at the cecum, with directional flow toward the rectum
    c. Begins at the rectum and ends at the cecum, with a directional flow toward the cecum
    d. Begins at the splenic flexure and ends at the hepatic flexure, with directional flow toward the sigmoid colon

27. *Micturition is _____.*

    a. Parasympathetic action to void urine
    b. Sympathetic action to increase retention of feces
    c. Movement of blood through the nephrons
    d. Restoration of blood acid-base balance

Answers are on pages 102–104.

28. *When stretch receptors signal that the bladder needs to empty, what muscle contracts?*

    a. Pectineus
    b. Coccygeus
    c. Pyramidalis
    d. Detrusor

29. *Cystitis is _____.*

    a. Inflammation of the medulla of the kidney
    b. Infection of the glomerulus
    c. Bladder infection
    d. Obstruction of the urethra

30. *Why might massage be contraindicated for those with renal insufficiency?*

    a. Massage causes increase in blood pressure
    b. Massage increases blood volume through the kidneys
    c. Massage spreads bacteria through the urinary system
    d. Massage increases the difficulty with incontinence

31. *Erectile tissue is able to become firmer because _____.*

    a. This tissue engorges with blood
    b. Muscles contract, stiffening the tissue
    c. The tissue absorbs water from the lymph
    d. Smooth muscles encircle the tissue, acting as a sphincter

32. *Thirty minutes into a relaxation massage a male client has an erection. What is the most logical reason for this response?*

    a. The client has been "sexualizing" the massage
    b. Erection is a parasympathetic response
    c. Stimulation of the skin shifts blood flow
    d. Activation of sympathetic reflexes triggers the response

33. *Which of the following secretes a lubricating fluid in the female external genitalia?*

    a. Fundus
    b. Bartholin gland
    c. Clitoris
    d. Symphysis pubis

34. *During sexual development in the female, which occurs last?*

    a. Hypothalamus matures
    b. Estradiol is produced
    c. Adrenal cortex hormone signals pubic hair growth
    d. Ovulation

35. *The alkaline nature of semen is to _____.*

    a. Stimulate orgasm
    b. Counteract the acid nature of vaginal fluid
    c. Thin the protective coating of the ovum
    d. Lubricate the ejaculatory duct

36. *If a female client is in the second trimester of a pregnancy, which of the following would most apply?*

    a. Massage will be most comfortable if it is given with the client prone
    b. Massage will be most comfortable if client is positioned on their side
    c. Massage of the feet is contraindicated
    d. Massage should focus most on lymphatic drainage

37. *During massage a lactating client experiences the letdown response. What would be the most likely cause?*

    a. Massage stimulates the release of oxytocin
    b. Massage stimulates the production of testosterone
    c. Massage decreases colostrum
    d. Massage decreases libido

38. *Which of the following sexually transmitted diseases has a bacterial origin?*

    a. Genital warts
    b. Herpes genitalis
    c. Gonorrhea
    d. Hepatitis B

39. *A 56-year old male client complains of difficulty voiding urine. What would be the most likely diagnosis from his physician?*

    a. Endometriosis
    b. *Trichomonas* vaginitis
    c. Bartholin cyst
    d. Benign prostatic hypertrophy

40. *A client is experiencing weakness and exhaustion; impaired concentration, memory, and performance; disturbed sleep; and emotional sweating. A complete physical has ruled out any existing pathology. Stress is indicated as a probable cause. Which of the following treatment plans would best reverse the stress response?*

    a. Massage to promote lymphatic drainage and stimulate arterial circulation
    b. Massage to support proper breathing function and reverse hyperventilation syndrome
    c. Massage to reduce scar tissue and prevent adhesions
    d. Massage to stimulate increase in heart rate and blood pressure

41. *A couple has experienced difficulties conceiving a third child. The doctors can find no reason for the difficulties. The male is a regular client. He asks if massage could be of help. The answer is yes. Which of the following justification statements is most logical?*

    a. Massage can assist in the success of sexual intercourse by encouraging adrenaline secretion
    b. Massage can increase the rate of ovulation by stimulating the hypothalamus to secrete follicle-stimulating hormone
    c. Massage can encourage more efficient homeostatic mechanism in the body, promoting general health, including fertility
    d. Massage can increase the levels of testosterone, prolactin, and progesterone, promoting ovulation

42. *A massage therapist feels restless on days off and finds it more difficult to sleep. What is the most logical reason for this phenomenon?*

    a. Providing massage usually promotes a parasympathetic response in both the client and the practitioner; on days when no massage is performed, the practitioner does not stimulate relaxation responses as effectively
    b. Providing massage is fatiguing; on days off the massage practitioner has more energy
    c. Providing massage interferes with natural entrainment responses, and on days off the practitioner is more in tune with biorhythms
    d. Providing massage increases adrenaline and other stimulating hormones and neurotransmitters; when this occurs, hyperventilation syndrome is common, resulting in restlessness and sleep disturbances

Answers are on pages 102–104.

Answers and Discussion

1. **a**
   Factual recall
   Rationale: Defining the terminology is necessary to answer the question. The question is the definition of breathing.

2. **d**
   Factual recall
   Rationale: The question describes the location of the septum. Make sure to know the location of all the structures listed.

3. **b**
   Application and concept identification
   Rationale: Each of the answers has to be analyzed both for correct information and in relationship to the question. Only answer b meets both criteria.

4. **d**
   Factual recall
   Rationale: The question defines alveoli. Always define the terminology and identify the location of the structures for questions of this type.

5. **a**
   Factual recall
   Rationale: The question describes a physiologic state and asks for how a structure would respond. All the terminology needs to be defined and understood in relation to the sympathetic state.

6. **b**
   Factual recall
   Rationale: The question is asking about anatomy in relationship to function. Since the phrenic nerve allows the diaphragm to function and the injury is below this area, breathing without assistance is possible.

7. **c**
   Factual recall
   Rationale: The question is about muscle function resulting in rib movement up and out, which creates the vacuum drawing air into the lungs.

8. **d**
   Application and concept identification
   Rationale: This question and the possible answers first require that the terminology be defined and the meaning of the question and answers interpreted. This is a common question type. Then the answers need to be analyzed to identify the correct answer. Tachypnea is fast breathing, which would increase oxygen levels, drop carbon dioxide levels, and trigger sympathetic dominance. This is a cause of hyperventilation syndrome.

9. **b**
   Clinical reasoning/synthesis
   Rationale: The facts are located in the question and in the textbook. Symptoms and treatment of asthma would need to be understood. This is true of any pathology before attempting to decide what benefit massage has to offer and to identify contraindications and need for referral. The possibilities offered in the possible answers must be analyzed for safe and effective application. The problem is bronchoconstriction, so answer a is incorrect. Answer b is correct. Both answers c and d would increase the problem.

10. **a**
    Factual recall
    Rationale: All the listed pathologies need to be defined and the one that is contagious identified.

11. **c**
    Application and concept identification
    Rationale: The question is asking for the physiologic interaction with massage, ANS, and breathing. The three wrong answers present information contrary to the identified effects of massage.

12. **b**
    Factual recall
    Rationale: Addictive behavior is related to stimulation of pleasure sensations.

13. **a**
    Factual recall
    Rationale: Defining the terminology and identifying the location of the structures are necessary to answer the question. The question describes the peritoneum.

14. **d**
    Factual recall
    Rationale: Digestive enzymes need to be identified in relation to the food groups they work on to choose the correct answer.

15. **b**
    Factual recall
    Rationale: Defining the terminology and identifying the location of the structures are necessary to answer the question. The question describes the rugae.

16. **c**
    Factual recall
    Rationale: Defining the terminology and identifying the location of the structures are necessary to answer the question. The question describes the duodenum.

17. **c**
Factual recall
Rationale: Defining the terminology and identifying the function of the structures are necessary to answer the question. The question describes the liver.

18. **a**
Factual recall
Rationale: Defining the terminology and function of the large intestine are necessary to answer the question.

19. **b**
Factual recall
Rationale: Defining the terminology and identifying the location and function of the structures are necessary to answer the question. The question describes the appendix.

20. **c**
Clinical reasoning/synthesis
Rationale: The answer is the correct justification for why massage would achieve the outcome of managing the symptoms listed. Each of the presented treatment plans must be analyzed for effectiveness and safety. All terms need to be defined and the statements interpreted before choosing the correct answer. Sympathetic dominance tends to aggravate digestive problems. Answer b is not a safe practice. Answer c is correct. Answer d includes supporting upper chest breathing, indicating sympathetic dominance, so the content in the answer is flawed.

21. **a**
Factual recall
Rationale: Defining the terminology is necessary to answer the question. The question describes protein.

22. **b**
Application and concept identification
Rationale: The question is asking for the connection between fats and hormone production.

23. **c**
Factual recall
Rationale: Defining the pathologic conditions is necessary to answer the question. The question describes cirrhosis.

24. **b**
Factual recall
Rationale: Defining the pathologic conditions is necessary to answer the question. The question describes hepatitis.

25. **d**
Factual recall
Rationale: Defining the pathologic conditions is necessary to answer the question. The question describes strangulated hernia.

26. **b**
Application and concept identification
Rationale: Stimulation of movement of fecal material through the large intestine may be assisted by massage that simulates the peristaltic action of the large intestine and flows along the same anatomic route.

27. **a**
Factual recall
Rationale: The terms need definition to identify the correct answer.

28. **d**
Factual recall
Rationale: The question is asking for a muscle function. All listed muscles need to be identified for location and function to correctly answer the question.

29. **c**
Factual recall
Rationale: The question is asking for a definition of a pathology. To identify the correct answer, the common diseases of the urinary system need to be learned. Medical terminology interpretation is helpful. Cyst- means bladder.

30. **b**
Application and concept identification
Rationale: The question asks for an effect of massage that may be contraindicated if a particular pathology is present. Renal insufficiency would make it difficult for the kidneys to handle increased blood volume.

31. **a**
Factual recall
Rationale: The correct answer explains the physiology of erectile tissue.

32. **b**
Application and concept identification
Rationale: The correct answer explains the physiology of the male erection in response to parasympathetic dominance.

33. **b**
Factual recall
Rationale: All the terms need to be defined to answer the question.

34. **d**
    Factual recall
    Rationale: Ovulation is the last to occur as the female sexually matures.

35. **b**
    Factual recall
    Rationale: The question asks for the reason for the pH of semen.

36. **b**
    Application and concept identification
    Rationale: An understanding of the stages of pregnancy, positioning of the client, and indications and contraindications for massage is required to answer the question.

37. **a**
    Application and concept identification
    Rationale: The terms need to be defined and an understanding of the relationship of oxytocin to massage and lactation is necessary.

38. **c**
    Factual recall
    Rationale: All the pathologies listed need to be defined to identify gonorrhea as the correct answer.

39. **d**
    Factual recall
    Rationale: All the pathologies listed need to be defined to identify benign prostatic hypertrophy as the correct answer.

40. **b**
    Clinical reasoning/synthesis
    Rationale: Based on the symptoms described in the question, the most logical cause is disrupted breathing function, which creates sympathetic dominance. The treatment described in answer b would address this situation best.

41. **c**
    Clinical reasoning/syntheses
    Rationale: The correct answer would provide correct justification for how massage may help some types of infertility conditions that are related to stress. Each answer needs to be analyzed for correct information in relationship to the outcome. Adrenaline does not promote decreased stress response. Massage has not been shown to affect follicle-stimulating hormone. Answer c is the correct answer. Massage has not been shown to affect the hormones listed, and these same hormones may inhibit ovulation.

42. **a**
    Clinical reasoning/synthesis
    Rationale: This question asks for a decision based on accumulated knowledge from textbooks in relation to massage practice and physiologic effects. The facts in the question indicated sympathetic autonomic nervous system activation. The correct answer would explain why this is so. Answer a is the most logical. Massage done correctly should not be excessively fatiguing. Massage promotes entrainment. Answer d is not logical.

SECTION

7. The practice of acupuncture involves _____.

   a. The stimulation of specific points along the
        body, usually by the insertion of tiny, solid
        needles
   b. The stimulation of specific points along the
        body, usually by the pressing of the thumb
        into the point
   c. The stimulation of broad points along the
        body, usually by accomplishing a series of
        ever-deepening compressive strokes
   d. Using counterirritation, such as scraping,
        cutting, or burning of skin, to relieve pain

8. Polarity therapy was created by _____.

   a. Dr. James B. Mennell
   b. Randolph Stone
   c. Wilhelm Reich
   d. Dr. Janet Travell

9. Henrick Ling was a noted _____.

   a. Physician who developed massage
        techniques for joint stiffness and wound
        healing
   b. Swedish writer who wrote De Medicina, a
        series of eight books covering the body of
        knowledge of the day
   c. Teacher who is credited with developing
        Swedish massage
   d. Physician credited with bringing massage to
        the scientific community

10. The National Certification Examination for Therapeutic Massage and Bodywork was first devised in _____.

    a. 1980
    b. 1992
    c. 1974
    d. 1998

11. One of the prominent reasons that Ling's work had a difficult time being accepted was because _____.

    a. He worked only with healthy people
    b. He used poetic and mystic language in his writings
    c. He based it on newly discovered knowledge of the circulation of the blood and lymph
    d. The primary focus was on gymnastics

12. What is the massage trend that developed in 1991 that supported acceptance for the benefits of massage?

    a. Increase in valid research
    b. Deregulation of massage education
    c. Decrease in influential women in the profession
    d. Resistance to integrating massage into traditional health care settings

Answers and Discussion

1. **d**
   Factual recall
   Rationale: The correct answer is the definition of professionalism.

2. **c**
   Factual recall
   Rationale: The question provides a example of age issues and the interpretation of professional touch. The entire issue of touch perceptions needs to be understood to answer the question.

3. **b**
   Application and concept identification
   Rationale: The question addresses the issue of how touch interaction can be experienced by an individual.

4. **b**
   Factual recall
   Rationale: The correct answer is the definition of culture.

5. **b**
   Factual recall
   Rationale: The various forms of touch need to be defined to identify touch technique and mechanical touch.

6. **a**
   Factual recall
   Rationale: The history of massage has a basis in the terminology and historical origins.

7. **a**
   Factual recall
   Rationale: The correct answer is a definition of acupuncture.

8. **b**
   Factual recall
   Rationale: It is important to remember historical figures who have contributed to the body of knowledge of massage and bodywork. While Randolph Stone is the correct answer to the question, the others also made significant contributions.

9. **c**
   Factual recall
   Rationale: It is important to remember historical figures who have contributed to the body of knowledge of massage and bodywork.

10. **b**
    Factual recall
    Rationale: It is important to remember historical events that have influenced massage and bodywork.

11. **b**
    Factual recall
    Rationale: It is important to remember historical events that have influenced massage and bodywork.

12. **a**
    Factual recall
    Rationale: It is important to remember historical events that have influenced massage and bodywork. Research currently is a major influence on the profession.

14

Professionalism and Legal Issues

Questions

1. *The knowledge base and practice parameters of a profession are called _____.*

   a. Scope of practice
   b. Informed consent
   c. Dual role
   d. Therapeutic relationship

2. *A massage professional becomes angry with a client who complains about personal problems during the massage. The massage practitioner is displaying _____.*

   a. Transference
   b. Therapeutic relationship
   c. Ethical behavior
   d. Countertransference

3. *A massage professional does not regularly drape all clients in a modest and professional manner. Which of the following best describes this conduct?*

   a. The massage professional practices a dual role
   b. The massage professional has breached a standard of practice
   c. The massage professional is involved in misuse of the scope of practice
   d. The massage professional needs additional training in draping

4. *A massage professional works with three main populations: athletes, those with chronic pain, and clients requiring stress management. The therapist uses a variety of methods. Which of the following best describes the massage application style being used?*

   a. Structural and postural approaches
   b. Applied kinesiology
   c. Integrated approaches
   d. Myofascial methods

5. *A massage professional has been working with a particular client for 12 months. Recently the client has been experiencing increasing difficulties with the family communications. The biggest problem is stress and tension between son and father. Discussions during massage are centered around solving this problem. Which of the following best describes this situation?*

   a. Massage professional is having difficulty maintaining informed consent
   b. Scope of practice violations, particularly with psychology, are occurring
   c. The client should be referred for either acupuncture or chiropractic
   d. The client is engaged in countertransference

6. *A client, a professional dancer, is basically healthy but is seeking massage to manage minor injury and support recovery. Which scope of practice description best describes these outcomes?*

    a. Wellness/normal function
    b. Health care services
    c. Dysfunction and athletic performance
    d. Illness/trauma

7. *A massage professional with entry-level training has been seeing a client recently diagnosed with diabetes. The massage professional is becoming more uncomfortable providing massage as the client displays more symptoms. What is occurring?*

    a. The massage professional is in a dual role now that the client is ill
    b. The client is more demanding of the professional
    c. The massage professional has failed to abide by the definition of massage
    d. The massage professional is functioning outside the personal scope of practice

8. *A massage professional is very careful to provide an informed consent process for each client and updates informed consent on a regular basis. Which of the following ethical principles is being followed?*

    a. Confidentiality
    b. Justice
    c. Proportionality
    d. Client autonomy and self-determination

9. *Taking a client's history and providing a physical assessment to develop a massage care plan is called a _____.*

    a. Needs assessment
    b. Brochure and policy statement
    c. Release of information
    d. Chart

10. *A massage professional has worked very hard to develop a policy statement and has included types of service offered, information on training and experience, appointment policies, client and practitioner expectations, sexual appropriateness, and recourse policy. What did the professional forget to include?*

    a. Number of appointments to meet therapeutic goals
    b. Fee structure
    c. Objective progress measurements
    d. Methods of clinical reasoning

11. *Which of the following is a violation of confidentiality?*

    a. Maintaining client records in a secure location
    b. Asking the client questions about work environment
    c. Approaching and speaking to a client in a restaurant
    d. Speaking to a client's chiropractor with appropriate releases

12. *Which of the following would be an appropriate disclosure to a client?*

    a. The fact that the massage professional has a cold
    b. Business financial concerns
    c. Discussion about a mutual acquaintance
    d. Marital difficulties

13. *A massage professional has been asked to work with a support group for persons with cerebral palsy. The therapist is well trained and has 7 years of experience but is uncomfortable with people with disabilities, especially if communication is problematic. Which of the following is grounds for refusal on the part of the massage professional?*

    a. Lack of skills
    b. Lack of peer support
    c. Inability to serve without bias
    d. Only wishes to work with females

14. *A massage professional with 15 years of experience but minimal continuing education is in charge of a massage clinic. A recent massage graduate has obtained a position at the clinic. The new graduate notices that his current skills, particularly in charting and critical thinking, are more sophisticated than those of his supervisor but is hesitant to discuss the issue. What is the best description for this situation?*

   a. Power differential
   b. Dual role
   c. Maintenance of professional environment
   d. Reciprocity

15. *Which of the following is the best example of transference?*

   a. A massage professional is biased toward a client due to political beliefs
   b. A massage professional is receiving small gifts from a client expressing affection
   c. A massage professional asks a client to attend a meeting about a nutritional product with him
   d. A client is angry with the massage professional for being late for the last three appointments

16. *Which of the following would be the best explanation for a client who is confused over an incident of becoming mildly sexually aware during the last massage?*

   a. The massage practitioner was sexualizing the massage
   b. The client was sexualizing the massage
   c. The client was experiencing parasympathetic sensations
   d. The massage practitioner was massaging erotic zones

17. *A massage practitioner made a practice of careful and modest draping during the massage, used low lighting and soft music to help clients relax, always locked the door to maintain privacy, provided informed consent, and maintained charting. Where is the greatest potential for ethical concerns?*

   a. Locked door
   b. Low lighting
   c. Soft music
   d. Confidential charting

18. *A massage professional is troubled over a client's responses during the last four massage sessions. There is nothing specific about the client's behavior, but something has changed in the client's response to the massage. What could be helpful to the massage professional?*

   a. Credentialing review with certification
   b. Managing intimacy issues
   c. Changing body language
   d. Decision making with peer support

19. *A client seems to interrupt often when the massage practitioner is attempting to gather information about the client's condition prior to the massage. The client often provides inaccurate information when asked questions. Where might the client need assistance in the communication process?*

   a. Formulating I-messages
   b. Listening
   c. Open-ended question
   d. Word choice

20. *A client informs a massage professional that another massage practitioner in the business is soliciting clients to move to a new private practice the therapist is starting. The massage professional knows that everyone in the massage practice signed a contract agreeing not to behave in this manner. After carefully consideration of the situation and discussion with a peer in a similar situation in another state, what is the next step in dealing with this type of unethical behavior of a peer?*

   a. Formal reporting
   b. Contacting a lawyer
   c. Talking with those involved
   d. Speaking to fellow workers

21. *Local legislation controlling the location of a business is _____.*

   a. Licensing
   b. Building codes
   c. DBA
   d. Zoning

Answers are on pages 114–115.

Answers and Discussion

1. **a**
Factual recall
Rationale: The question is the definition of scope of practice. As with all of these types of questions, all the terms need to be defined to understand and answer the question.

2. **d**
Application and concept identification
Rationale: The question gives an example of countertransference. As with all of these types of questions, all the terms need to be defined to understand and answer the question. The behavior of the massage professional described in the question needs to be compared to the definition.

3. **b**
Application and concept identification
Rationale: The question provides an example of breach of a standard of practice. The terms need to be defined.

4. **c**
Application and concept identification
Rationale: The question addresses various approaches to massage and bodywork. A description of the population and indication of application of a variety of methods indicate that this professional uses an integrated approach.

5. **b**
Application and concept identification
Rationale: The question provides an example of a breach in scope of practice. To identify the correct answer, all the terms need to be defined and understood in relation to the behavior.

6. **c**
Factual recall
Rationale: The question provides an example of the scope of practice for working with those with complex situations but who are not ill.

7. **d**
Application and concept identification
Rationale: The question gives an example and the correct answer would explain a logical reason why the practitioner is uncomfortable. This is not a dual role, transference, or even a technical breach of scope of practice for massage, but the personal scope of practice is affected since the massage professional did not receive enough training to address this complex disease condition.

8. **d**
Factual recall
Rationale: The ethical principles need to be defined to identify the correct answer.

9. **a**
Factual recall
Rationale: The question is the definition of a needs assessment.

10. **b**
Factual recall
Rationale: The question lists all the components of a policy statement except fee structure. The wrong answers are part of either a treatment plan or a clinical reasoning process.

11. **c**
Application and concept identification
Rationale: The correct answer would indicate that confidentiality has been breached. The three wrong answers are examples of maintaining confidentiality.

12. **a**
Application and concept identification
Rationale: First the term disclosure needs to be defined. The correct example can be identified. Only information that would directly affect the massage interaction is to be disclosed. The three wrong answers are examples of inappropriate conversation with a client.

13. **c**
Application and concept identification
Rationale: The question asks for a rationale for the right of refusal. The only answer that is logical based on the facts in the question is answer c.

14. **a**
Application and concept identification
Rationale: The question gives an example of the power differential but in a different context than the examples in the textbook. The other terms, once defined, would not be logical in relation to the facts of the question.

15. **b**
Application and concept identification
Rationale: First transference needs to be defined and then compared to the examples provided in the possible answers. Answer a is countertransference, answer b is correct, answer c is dual role, and answer d is justifiable anger, not transference.

16. **c**
Application and concept identification
Rationale: The most logical answer is answer c.
The facts of the question indicate that the client
is confused over the sensations and indicate no
intentional acts by either party.

17. **a**
Factual recall
Rationale: Locking the door is entrapment.

18. **d**
Application and concept identification
Rationale: The question provides an example of a
situation in which peer support is helpful in
ethical decision making. The three wrong
answers would indicate that the professional has
decided what the problem is, but the question
indicates otherwise. Peer support and ethical
decision making are helpful in identifying the
area of concern and developing plans to rectify
the situation.

19. **b**
Factual recall
Rationale: The question gives examples of
listening difficulties.

20. **c**
Factual recall
Rationale: The question is asking for the steps in
dealing with peer behavior.

21. **d**
Factual recall
Rationale: This question is representative of how
information about credentialing and legal
operation can be tested. The terms need to be
defined to answer the question.

15

Medical Terminology for Professional Record Keeping

Questions

1. *Record keeping for clients involves* _____.

   a. Charting each session of the ongoing process
   b. Having the client fill out a general information packet
   c. Written record of intake procedures, informed consent, needs assessments, recording of each session, and release of information
   d. Filing each piece of information received from physicians, insurance companies, or payments received from clients

2. *Charting can be defined as* _____.

   a. A record of each payment made by the client
   b. A record of the time spent with each client
   c. A written record of the intake procedure
   d. The ongoing process of recording each session

3. *All goals must be quantified, meaning* _____.

   a. That they are achievable
   b. That they are measured in terms of objective criteria
   c. How they will be done
   d. What they will cost

4. *The purpose of gathering a database is to* _____.

   a. Gather information on which to build the professional interaction, establish client goals, and develop a plan for achieving them
   b. Develop a comprehensive knowledge base of medical terms to be able to reason clinically and chart effectively
   c. Develop procedures for writing records and the ways to use various forms
   d. Set achievable goals and outline a general plan

5. *A database consists of* _____.

   a. Charts on the actual session
   b. All the information available that contributes to therapeutic interaction
   c. The client's description of the problem
   d. Goals that are quantified and qualified as well as functionally oriented.

6. *The purpose of assessment is to* _____.

   a. Provide methods to correct deviations from the norm
   b. Identify effective functioning in order to eliminate massage to that area
   c. Do a visual and functional assessment but not a palpation assessment
   d. Identify effective functioning and deviations from the norm

7. *Which of the following is a quantified outcome goal?*

   a. Client will be able to increase range of motion of the lateral flexion of the cervical area by 15 degrees

   b. Client will be able to resume normal work activities

   c. Client will be reassessed in 12 sessions

   d. Client will recover ability to play golf

8. *In order to analyze the data gathered during the assessment, one must _____.*

   a. Increase mechanical application of skills for application of the treatment plan

   b. Generate quantifiable goals and methods to achieve client goals

   c. Consider the information based on examination, investigation, and analysis in relation to outcomes

   d. Compare information to generalized norms and protocols for treatment

9. *The treatment plan _____.*

   a. Is an exact protocol developed by client and practitioner

   b. Is a fluid guideline developed by client and practitioner

   c. Must be complete at the end of the first session and not revised

   d. Must be complete before the massage begins, since information gathered during the massage is not relevant

10. *Problem-oriented medical records including SOAP require that _____.*

   a. The qualified goals and the outcome of the massage be noted on the record

   b. The facts, possibilities, logical consequences of cause and effect, and impact on people be noted on the record

   c. The results of palpation assessment but not the client history be recorded

   d. Only the interventions be noted on the record

11. *Which of the following would be recorded in the objective data section of a SOAP note?*

   a. Client states she has interrupted sleep

   b. Client is currently taking melatonin

   c. Observation and palpation indicate upper chest breathing

   d. Client wishes to have weekly appointments

12. *The most important area in terms of determining future intervention procedures based on results is _____.*

   a. S: subjective—what the client states

   b. O: objective—what was observed from assessment and examination

   c. A: analysis—what worked/did not work

   d. P: plan—what client wants to work on and what needs to be done during the next session

13. *P (plan) part of SOAP should include _____.*

   a. Client medication history

   b. Client self-care

   c. Key symptoms

   d. Relation of outcomes to goals

14. *The purpose of using a clinical reasoning model is _____.*

   a. To be able to think through an intervention process and justify the effectiveness of a therapeutic interaction

   b. To provide a primary means of effectively supporting diagnosis to other health care professionals

   c. To integrate all the modalities and techniques into a user-friendly charting process for all to understand

   d. To provide a framework for the client charting protocols and data collection

15. *A client presents a physician referral that states that only general massage with light pressure is to be used due to a recent angioplasty. The suffix in angioplasty means _____.*

   a. Tumor

   b. Enlargement

   c. Surgical repair

   d. Disease

16. *Reading the history, the massage professional sees that the client lists having myalgia. Which of the following defines myalgia?*

    a. Muscle condition
    b. Spine pain
    c. Muscle pain
    d. Muscle paralysis

17. *While reviewing a file on a client referred from another massage therapist, the massage professional finds information in the SOAP charting that indicates that applications of effleurage to the legs resulted in vasodilation. Which body system was directly affected?*

    a. Cardiovascular
    b. Urinary
    c. Immune
    d. Digestive

18. *What needs to be done to develop a valid analysis of massage benefits in a SOAP chart?*

    a. Completion of a treatment plan
    b. Pre- and postassessment procedures
    c. Prior development of a problem-oriented medical record
    d. Dates of reassessment

19. *A massage professional lists reducing neuritis as a long-term client goal in the treatment plan. Which of the following describes the outcome?*

    a. Provide relief from intestinal spasm
    b. Provide a decrease in joint mobility
    c. Produce an increase in nerve conduction
    d. Provide a decrease in nerve inflammation

20. *Where would a massage professional record this statement on a SOAP note: "Palpation identified mild scoliosis"?*

    a. S
    b. O
    c. A
    d. P

Answers and Discussion

1. **c**
   Factual recall
   Rationale: The answer describes record-keeping responsibilities.

2. **d**
   Factual recall
   Rationale: The correct answer is the definition of charting.

3. **b**
   Factual recall
   Rationale: The correct answer is the definition of a quantifiable goal.

4. **a**
   Factual recall
   Rationale: The correct answer describes the use of a database.

5. **b**
   Factual recall
   Rationale: The correct answer describes the components of a database.

6. **d**
   Factual recall
   Rationale: The correct answer describes the reason for assessment.

7. **a**
   Application and concept identification
   Rationale: First a quantified outcome goal must be defined and then the possible answers analyzed for which one fits the criteria. Two of the wrong answers are examples of qualified goals.

8. **c**
   Factual recall
   Rationale: The correct answer describes the proper reason for data analysis.

9. **b**
   Factual recall
   Rationale: The correct answer is a definition of a treatment plan. The incorrect answers all present inaccurate information.

10. **b**
    Factual recall
    Rationale: The correct answer describe the contents of proper charting.

11. **c**
    Application and concept identification
    Rationale: A type of objective data is information collected from assessment, as described in the correct answer. Answers a and b are subjective data, and answer d is information for the treatment plan.

12. **c**
    Application and concept identification
    Rationale: The decision-making process is being described in the question, and this happens during the analysis.

13. **b**
    Factual recall
    Rationale: The answer describes data recorded as part of the plan.

14. **a**
    Application and concept identification
    Rationale: The wrong answers are reasons for record keeping. Clinical reasoning is a process of thinking.

15. **c**
    Factual recall
    Rationale: This is a common approach to question development about medical terminology.

16. **c**
    Factual recall
    Rationale: This is a common approach to question development about medical terminology.

17. **a**
    Factual recall
    Rationale: This is a common approach to question development about medical terminology.

18. **b**
    Application and concept identification
    Rationale: The question asks for components of analysis. Required is a pre- and postassessment to determine results.

19. **d**
    Application and concept identification
    Rationale: Knowledge of medical terminology is required to interpret the question. Neuritis is nerve inflammation.

20. **b**
    Factual recall
    Rationale: This is a common approach to question development about SOAP charting.

16

Scientific Art of Therapeutic Massage

Questions

1. Science is defined as _____.
   a. Knowing something without going through a conscious process of thinking
   b. The ability to pay attention to a specific area and maintain an unconscious focus and intent
   c. The intellectual process of using all mental and physical resources available to better understand, explain, and predict normal and unusual natural phenomena
   d. Craft, skill, and technique that enable a person to monitor and adjust involuntary or subconscious responses

2. Centering is _____.
   a. A craft, skill, technique, and talent
   b. The ability to pay attention and maintain specific focus
   c. Knowing something without going through a conscious process of thinking
   d. The objective researching of a concept to see if it is valid

3. The purpose of valid research in massage is to _____.
   a. Generate more questions about massage
   b. Objectively research the physiologic process
   c. Subjectively research the massage process
   d. Justify massage as an art

4. The techniques of therapeutic massage provide manual external sensory stimulation. Which of the following would be a good example?
   a. Entrainment
   b. Rubbing ~ only manual stimulation choice
   c. Centering
   d. Breathing

5. Most agree that the effects of massage can be explained by two categories: _____.
   a. Reflexive and mechanical methods
   b. Centering and intuition
   c. Art and experimentation
   d. Art and intuition

6. Which methods directly affect (stimulate) the nervous system?
   a. Mechanical methods
   b. Circulatory methods
   c. Reflexive methods
   d. Connective tissue methods

7. *We now know that biochemicals are responsible for most problems in behavior, mood, and perception of stress and pain. Which of the following is an example of this type of problem?*

   a. Anxiety
   b. Obstructive sleep apnea
   c. Eczema
   d. Farsightedness

8. *Massage can increase a person's fine motor movements such as handwriting. Which neurotransmitter is influenced?*

   a. Serotonin
   b. Oxytocin
   c. Dopamine → *increases (motor fine skill)*
   d. Growth hormone

   define all

9. *Massage has been demonstrated to reduce some people's craving for food and/or reduce hunger. Which neurotransmitter is responsible?*

   a. Epinephrine
   b. Serotonin
   c. Dopamine
   d. Norepinephrine

   define

10. *If I wanted my employees to be more attentive, I would do massage for _____.*

    a. 5 minutes
    b. 45 minutes
    c. 15 minutes
    d. 60 minutes

11. *Connectedness and intimacy in massage are most likely the results of an increased level of _____.*

    a. Cortisol
    b. Endorphins
    c. Serotonin
    d. Oxytocin

    define

    worth neurotransmitters ?

12. *Massage has been shown to reduce levels of _____, which decreases sympathetic arousal.*

    a. Cortisol
    b. Oxytocin
    c. Growth hormone
    d. Enkephalins

    define - cortisol

    ?

13. *A client states a goal of wanting to relax and complains of having headaches, gastrointestinal problems, and high blood pressure. The client is likely to be experiencing _____.*

    a. An excessive parasympathetic output
    b. An excessive sympathetic output
    c. An entrainment process normalization
    d. Sleep deprivation

14. *Hans Selye described body responses to stress in three stages. The middle stage is called _____.*

    a. Alarm reaction
    b. Exhaustion reaction
    c. Resistance reaction
    d. Entrainment reaction

15. *What is the general term used to describe the initial activation of the sympathetic nervous system?*

    a. Alarm
    b. Stress
    c. Entrapment
    d. Entrainment - *define*

16. *A person experiencing fluid retention, muscle weakness, vertigo, hypersensitivity, fatigue, weight gain, and breakdown in connective tissue most likely has _____.*

    ?.

    a. Test anxiety
    b. Long-term high blood levels of cortisol
    c. First-stage/alarm reaction
    d. Conservation withdrawal

17. *What type of massage has been demonstrated to be most helpful for a client who has reached the exhaustive reaction phase of stress and been there for over 6 months?*

    a. Several appointments over 1 month using 15 minutes of tapotement and shaking
    b. A massage using pulling and pressing with light pressure for weekly sessions for 3 months
    c. A massage that primarily focuses on long slow strokes, broad-based compression, and rocking for weekly appointments for 6 months
    d. A staccato, fast deep pressure during weekly massage for 6 months

18. *Parasympathetic patterns are _____.*

    a. Restorative—adrenaline is secreted, mobility is decreased, and the bronchioles are constricted
    b. Physical activity is curtailed, digestion and elimination are increased, and the bronchioles are constricted
    c. Physical activity is increased, pupils are dilated, saliva secretion is stopped, and stomach secretion is increased
    d. Restorative—heartbeat speeds up, bladder delays emptying, and saliva secretion increases

19. *If a conservation withdrawal pattern is apparent, it can be the result of _____.*

    a. Intense negative experiences
    b. Synchronization to a rhythm
    c. A reflex response
    d. Reduction of air impingement

20. *In the human body, what initiates entrainment?*

    a. Digestive glands
    b. Autonomic nerves
    c. Brain
    d. Biologic oscillators

21. *A client becomes very relaxed in response to the music and the rhythm of the strokes used during the massage session. What has occurred?*

    a. Mechanical effects
    b. Circulation decrease
    c. Entrainment
    d. Client education

22. *An altered state of consciousness can be achieved by massage. For its most therapeutic effect, the massage must be how long?*

    a. 5 minutes
    b. 10 minutes
    c. 90 minutes
    d. 45 minutes

23. *State-dependent memory can be triggered by massage because _____.*

    a. The massage triggers, through movement or pressure, a stored pattern and stored release of chemical codes of emotions
    b. The massage presentation of stimuli teaches the body to manage more efficiently with sympathetic stress responses
    c. The massage itself influences the course of the memory, even if the massage is not specific to that memory
    d. Massage influences biologic oscillators such as the heart and thalamus, which sets rhythm patterns opposite the memory pattern

24. *There are three main types of proprioceptors: muscle spindles, tendon organs, and _____.*

    a. Cervical/lumbar plexus
    b. Spinal nerves
    c. Joint kinesthetic receptors
    d. Sphincter muscles

25. *A client gets a cramp in the hamstring when stretching too quickly. Which reflex prompted the action?*

    a. Stretch reflex
    b. Hooke's reflex
    c. Flexor reflex
    d. Extensor reflex

26. *The most common bodywork technique that involves the tendon reflex is _____.*

    a. Muscle toning
    b. Postisometric relaxation
    c. Acupuncture
    d. Counterirritation

27. *What reflex is involved in maintaining balance?*

    a. Flexor reflex
    b. Withdrawal reflex
    c. Tendon reflex
    d. Crossed extensor reflex

28. *The Arndt-Shultz law states: Weak stimuli activate physiologic processes; very strong stimuli inhibit them. What are the implications for massage?*

a. Massage is a strong sensory stimulation
b. Techniques have to be intense to produce responses
c. It is difficult to figure out if a pain originates from a joint or surrounding tissue
d. To encourage a specific response, use gentler methods; to shut off the response, use deeper methods

29. *The law of facilitation states: When an impulse has passed through a certain set of neurons to the exclusion of others one time, it will tend to take the same course on a future occasion, and each time it travels this path the resistance will be smaller. What are the implications for massage?*

a. If a sensory receptor is activated, it will respond in a certain way
b. Methods must override a sensation to produce a response
c. The body likes sameness; after a pattern has been established, less stimulation is required to activate the response
d. For a massage method to change a sensory perception, the intensity of the method must match and then exceed the existing sensation

30. *Some methods of massage affect the "ground substance." These include skin rolling, gliding strokes, and _____.* *define all*

a. Abrupt compression
b. Tapotement
c. Petrissage
d. Shaking

31. *The best way to increase arterial flow circulation enhancement during massage is _____.*

a. A 50-minute massage using effleurage but not heavy pressure
b. A 45-minute compressive massage against the arteries proximal to the heart and moving in a distal direction
c. A 50-minute massage using short pumping effleurage and gliding toward the heart
d. A 30-minute massage emphasizing gliding strokes to passive/active joint movement distal to proximal

32. *Gate control theory is _____.*

a. Reduction of perception of a sensation of a sensory receptor by adaptation
b. Control of homeostasis by alteration of tissue or function
c. A method of teaching the body to deal with stress
d. The hypothesis that painful stimuli can be prevented from reaching higher levels of the CNS by stimulating lower sensory nerves

33. *The gallbladder 30 acupuncture point location correlates with which of the following motor points?*

a. Triceps
b. Gastrocnemius
c. Gluteus maximus
d. Brachioradialis

34. *The triple heater meridian location corresponds with which nerve?*

a. Ulnar nerve
b. Tibial nerve
c. Sciatic nerve
d. Lateral plantar nerve

35. *Traditional chakra locations correspond to _____.*

a. Oxytocin
b. Arndt–Schulz law
c. Trigger points
d. Autonomic nerve plexuses

Answers and Discussion

1. **c**
   Factual recall
   Rationale: The correct answer is a definition of science.

2. **b**
   Factual recall
   Rationale: The correct answer is a definition of centering.

3. **b**
   Factual recall
   Rationale: Research objectively validates massage.

4. **b**
   Factual recall
   Rationale: Only rubbing provides manual stimulation.

5. **a**
   Factual recall
   Rationale: This question is testing terminology knowledge.

6. **c**
   Factual recall
   Rationale: The terms all need to be defined to answer the question.

7. **a**
   Factual recall
   Rationale: The question states a fact and then asks for the correct disorder. Anxiety is a mood disorder.

8. **c**
   Factual recall
   Rationale: The question is an example of how massage affects physiology. Information about neurotransmitter function is also required. Dopamine coordinates fine motor movement, and research shows dopamine availability increases with massage.

9. **b**
   Factual recall
   Rationale: The question is an example of how massage affects physiology. Information about neurotransmitter function is also required. Serotonin is involved with satiety, and availability increases with massage.

10. **c**
    Factual recall
    Rationale: The question is an example of how massage affects physiology. Information about neurotransmitter function is also required. Norepinephrine increases during the first 15 minutes of massage.

11. **d**
    Factual recall
    Rationale: The question is an example of how massage affects physiology. Information about neurotransmitter function is also required. Oxytocin availability increases with massage and is implicated in bonding.

12. **a**
    Factual recall
    Rationale: The question is an example of how massage affects physiology. Information about neurotransmitter function is also required. Cortisol decreases with a 30-minute or longer massage, which increases parasympathetic dominance.

13. **b**
    Application and concept identification
    Rationale: The question asks for a correlation between relaxation, the sympathetic symptoms displayed, and a massage outcome.

14. **c**
    Factual recall
    Rationale: Knowledge of the stages of the stress response is being tested. Entrainment is not part of the stress response.

15. **a**
    Factual recall
    Rationale: Terminology is being assessed by the question and possible answers. All terms need to be defined to answer the question.

16. **b**
    Application and concept identification
    Rationale: Answers a and c indicate an adrenaline response. The symptoms provided in the question indicate resistance response and the result of long-term exposure to cortisol. Answer d is a parasympathetic response pattern.

17. **c**
Clinical reasoning/synthesis
Rationale: The facts provided in the question are: long-term stress and a breakdown in adaptive capacity (exhaustion). Textbook facts would provide additional information about long-term cortisol effects, indications, and contraindications. Since the body is overstressed, care needs to be taken that the massage does not add excessive stress to the system. The wrong answers either strain the system or do not provide for a long enough intervention.

18. **b**
Factual recall
Rationale: The correct answer describes parasympathetic functions. Answer d uses terminology incorrectly.

19. **a**
Factual recall
Rationale: This is the emergency response of the parasympathetic system.

20. **d**
Factual recall
Rationale: The terms need to be defined to understand the connection between entrainment and the rhythms produced by biologic oscillators.

21. **c**
Application and concept identification
Rationale: The question asks for the reason for a physiologic response to massage and music in relation to the rhythm, which indicates an entrainment effect.

22. **d**
Factual recall
Rationale: It takes 45 minutes for the ANS to make a state change and allow for 15 minutes of effect.

23. **a**
Application and concept identification
Rationale: State-dependent memory is a conditioned response pattern that can be triggered by massage.

24. **c**
Factual recall
Rationale: This is a terminology question. All terms need to be defined to identify the correct answer.

25. **a**
Factual recall
Rationale: This is a terminology question. All terms need to be defined to identify the correct answer. There is no such thing as a Hooke's reflex but there is a Hooke's neurologic law. This misuse of terminology is a common strategy for developing wrong answers.

26. **b**
Application and concept identification
Rationale: The question asks for the physiologic mechanism responsible for the effect of a massage method. All the terms need to be defined to identify the correct answer.

27. **d**
Factual recall
Rationale: The question defines crossed extensor reflex.

28. **d**
Application and concept identification
Rationale: Neurologic laws identify consistent patterns of function. Applications of massage need to operate within this structure to have desired outcomes. Read the law carefully, interpret the terminology, and then project application to massage. Answer a is incorrect because massage stimulation can be either strong or weak. Technique does not have to be intense to produce a response. Answer c speaks to an entirely different neurologic law.

29. **c**
Application and concept identification
Rationale: Neurologic laws identify consistent patterns of function. Applications of massage need to operate within this structure to have desired outcomes. Read the law carefully, interpret the terminology, and then project application to massage. The law of facilitation speaks to the conservation of energy by repetition of response.

30. **c**
Factual recall
Rationale: Massage applications need to be defined as to effect on the ground substance of connective tissue.

31. **b**

    Application and concept identification
    Rationale: The question is an example of many different questions that can be written based on application of massage and bodywork methods to affect a body system. The information base in this question includes textbook data about the circulatory system and massage approaches to influence it. Answers a, c, and d are more focused on venous circulation.

32. **d**

    Factual recall
    Rationale: The correct answer defines gate control.

33. **c**

    Factual recall
    Rationale: This is an example of the type of question that correlates Eastern and Western theories in bodywork.

34. **a**

    Factual recall
    Rationale: This is an example of the type of question that correlates Eastern and Western theories in bodywork.

35. **d**

    Factual recall
    Rationale: This is an example of the type of question that correlates Eastern and Western theories in bodywork.

17

Indications and Contraindications for Therapeutic Massage

Questions

1. *A contraindication means an approach could be harmful. Which of the following is **not** a type of contraindication?*

   a. Support of a treatment modality other than massage

   b. General avoidance of an application—do not perform any massage techniques (person severely bruised over entire body)

   c. Regional avoidance of an application—do massage but avoid a particular area (person has broken foot)

   d. Application with caution—do massage with supervision but carefully select method, duration, and frequency

2. *Which of the following is **not** a general benefit of massage?*

   a. Improvement in circulation

   b. Enhanced elimination

   c. Inhibition of homeostasis

   d. Increased levels of endorphins

3. *Massage therapy benefits conditions by encouraging the body through the phases involved in rehabilitation, restoration, and _____ of anatomic and physiologic function.*

   a. Secretion

   b. Normalization

   c. Control

   d. Circulation

4. *A client is in the exhaustion phase of the general adaptation response. When one is considering a treatment plan for massage, which of the following is not appropriate?*

   a. Ability of the client to expend energy for active change

   b. The availability of support and resources during change process

   c. Practitioner must have appropriate knowledge and skills

   d. Completing outcomes in ten sessions or less

5. *Condition management involves the use of massage methods to support clients who cannot undergo a therapeutic change who but wish to be as effective as possible within an existing set of circumstances. Which of the following is an example of condition management?*

   a. Managing the existing physical compensation patterns
   b. Assisting the client through learning to walk again
   c. Restoring a client's range of motion to preinjury state
   d. Using massage to help a client feel better about self and to change jobs

6. *A client enters the massage room complaining of a bad back from working at the computer. There are no stated contraindications. This is a stage one dysfunction. The client wants to reverse the condition. Which approach is the best process?*

   a. Refer to low-back specialist
   b. Therapeutic change
   c. Condition management
   d. Palliative care

7. *Which of the following people may require only palliative care from a massage therapist?*

   a. An athlete with a sprained ankle RICG
   b. A 48-year-old female with a broken arm
   c. A man with terminal cancer
   d. A pregnant woman in the first trimester

8. *The definition of health is _____.*

   a. Prepathologic state
   b. Homeostatic and restorative body mechanisms can no longer adapt
   c. Anatomic and physiologic functioning limits
   d. Optimal functioning with freedom from disease or abnormal processes

9. *Pathology can be best defined as _____.*

   a. The in-between state of not healthy but not sick
   b. Anatomic and physiologic functioning limits
   c. The study of disease
   d. Processes of inflammatory tissue repair

10. *Which of the following statements is most correct?*

    a. The body has no actual anatomic or physiologic functioning limits
    b. The body has only anatomic functioning limits
    c. The body has only physiologic functioning limits
    d. The body has anatomic and physiologic functioning limits

11. *Disease conditions are usually defined, diagnosed, and identified by signs and symptoms. A sign is _____.*

    a. Subjective abnormalities felt only by the patient
    b. Objective abnormalities seen or measured by someone other than the patient
    c. A dysfunctional process noted by the patient
    d. An environmental situation described by the patient

12. *Homeostasis can be defined as _____.*

    a. The process of counterbalancing a defect in body structure or function
    b. A group of signs and symptoms
    c. The relative constancy of the body's internal environment
    d. The subjective abnormalities felt by the patient

13. *The general adaptation syndrome (body's response to stress) _____.*

    a. Is always a preexisting condition
    b. Involves three stages: alarm, resistance, and exhaustion
    c. Involves three stages: inflammatory response, swelling, and pain
    d. Is a genetic factor

14. *The inflammatory response can occur to any tissue injury. This response has four signs: redness, swelling, pain, and _____.*

    a. Stickiness
    b. Liquid
    c. Heat
    d. Mucus

What is palliative care

15. *What is it called when new cells are similar to those that they replace?*

    a. Egestion
    b. Fibrosis
    c. Inflammation
    d. Regeneration

16. *Massage has been shown to slow formation of scar tissue and helps keep scar tissue pliable. This assists the healing process by _____.*

    a. Blocking the action of antihistamines
    b. Counterbalancing the defect in the body
    c. Promoting regeneration and keeping replacement to a minimum
    d. Keeping the functioning energy reserves in place

17. *Therapeutic inflammation can be accomplished most effectively through _____.*

    a. Deep frictioning and connective tissue stretching
    b. Gliding
    c. Effleurage
    d. Tapotement and rapid compression

18. *Therapeutic inflammation is best utilized in situations _____.*

    a. In which there is a compromised immune function
    b. Resolving a fibrotic connective tissue dysfunction
    c. In which active inflammation is already present
    d. In which a condition like fibromyalgia exists

19. *The generally accepted definition of chronic pain is _____.*

    a. A symptom of a disease condition or a temporary aspect of medical treatment
    b. Pain frequently experienced by clients who have had a limb removed
    c. Pain that persists or recurs for indefinite periods, usually longer than 6 months
    d. Pain that often subsides with or without therapy

20. *Which of the following is a description of burning pain?*

    a. Short-lived but intense and easily localized
    b. Constant but not well localized
    c. Slow to develop, lasts longer, and less accurately localized
    d. Blood supply to the muscle is occluded, and contraction causes pain

21. *The origin of pain can be somatic or visceral. Somatic pain is defined as _____.*

    a. Pain from only stimulation of receptors in the skin
    b. Pain from only stimulation of receptors in the skeletal muscles, joints, or tendons
    c. Pain resulting from only stimulation of receptors in the internal organs
    d. Pain arising from stimulation of receptors in the skin, skeletal muscles, joints, tendons, and fascia

22. *If a client is experiencing pain in a surface area away from the stimulated organ, this is termed _____.*

    a. Muscle pain
    b. Referred pain
    c. Deep pain
    d. Acute pain

23. *Neck pain on the right side can be indicative of referred pain from what organs?*

    a. Appendix and kidney
    b. Colon and bladder
    c. Heart and lungs
    d. Liver and gallbladder

24. *Lung and diaphragm pain may be referred to which cutaneous area?*

    a. Left side of the neck
    b. Right side of the chest
    c. Right side of the neck
    d. In the hip girdle area

Answers are on pages 134–136.

25. *Intervention is different for managing acute versus chronic pain. Acute pain is managed _____.*

    a. With inhibitory methods
    b. Using aggressive rehabilitation approach
    c. Less invasively and focused to support current healing process
    d. By compression on a nerve in a bony structure

26. *Nerve impingement syndromes occur primarily in plexus areas. A person experiencing an impingement in the cervical plexus would have _____.*

    a. Shoulder pain, chest pain, arm pain, wrist pain, and hand pain
    b. Low-back discomfort with a belt distribution of pain as well as pain in lower abdomen, genitals, and thigh
    c. Gluteal pain, leg pain, genital pain, and foot pain
    d. Headaches, neck pain, and breathing difficulties

27. *Sacral plexus nerve impingement is indicated by _____.*

    a. Gluteal pain, leg pain, genital pain, and foot pain
    b. Headaches, neck pain, and breathing difficulties
    c. Shoulder pain, chest pain, arm pain, wrist pain, and hand pain
    d. Low-back discomfort with a belt distribution of pain and with pain in lower abdomen, genitals, thigh, and medial lower leg

28. *The most effective massage methods to work on impingement syndromes are _____.*

    a. Tapotement and shaking
    b. Muscle energy and lengthening
    c. Rapid deep compression
    d. Friction

29. *Regional contraindications are _____.*

    a. Those that require a physician's evaluation to rule out serious underlying conditions before any massage
    b. Present when health is the optimal functioning goal
    c. In effect when a client is in the in-between state of "not healthy" but also "not sick"
    d. Those that relate to a specific area of the body

30. *The difference between benign tumors and malignant tumors is _____.*

    a. Early detection is easier for benign tumors
    b. Malignant tumors are bigger
    c. Benign tumors remain localized within the tissue from which they arise; malignant tumors tend to spread to other regions of the body
    d. Benign tumors cannot grow rapidly

31. *Massage and medication have three general processes in common: they stimulate a body process, they replace a chemical in the body, and _____.*

    a. They work on a cure for the problem
    b. They work from a pathology base
    c. They inhibit a body process
    d. They remove cellular debris

32. *What occurs when medication and massage both stimulate the same process?*

    a. Antagonism
    b. Synergism
    c. Metastasis
    d. Impingement

33. *What is the major reason that massage practitioners need to be aware of endangerment sites?*

    a. These are soft areas that are unable to tolerate any pressure or movement

    b. They may be a sign of a life-threatening disorder

    c. The remaining proximal portions of sensory nerves are exposed here

    d. These areas are not well protected by muscle or connective tissue, so deep sustained pressure could damage vessels, nerves, or other structures

34. *Intractable pain is _____.*

    a. Cutaneous distribution of spinal nerve sensations

    b. A diffuse, localized discomfort that persists for indefinite periods

    c. Chronic pain that persists even when treatment is provided

    d. An abnormality in a body function that threatens well-being

35. *Predisposing conditions that may make the development of disease more likely by the client than by another person are called _____.*

    a. Metastasis

    b. Pathology

    c. Signs

    d. Risk factors

36. *Objective abnormalities that can be seen or measured by someone other than the client are _____.*

    a. Stress

    b. State-dependent memory

    c. Signs

    d. Pain

37. *The functions of the most abundant tissue of the body include support, structure, space, stabilization, and scar formation. What is this tissue?*

    a. Connective tissue

    b. Visceral tissue

    c. Bone marrow

    d. Fibrotic tissue

38. *A client is taking an anticoagulant. Which of the follow would be contraindicated?*

    a. Resting stoke

    b. Friction

    c. Muscle energy

    d. Rocking

39. *Which of the following is contraindicated for application of deep sustained compression?*

    a. Lymph nodes

    b. Trigger points

    •c. Dermatomes

    d. Ground substance

40. *A doctor referral is indicated if the _____.*

    a. Client has mild edema in the lower legs after a plane flight

    b. Client complains about care at the local outpatient client

    c. Client bruises easily

    d. Client is beginning a new medication

#38 anticoagulant ↳ blood thinner

? dERmatomEs

Answers and Discussion

1. **a**
   Factual recall
   Rationale: The three wrong answers are all correct examples of types of contraindications. This question is an example of how the correct answer is wrong information. Read questions written in this form very carefully.

2. **c**
   Factual recall
   Rationale: This question is another example of when the correct answer is wrong information. In this question massage does everything but produce inhibition of homeostasis.

3. **b**
   Factual recall
   Rationale: This is a terminology question. All of the terms need to be defined to correctly answer the question.

4. **d**
   Clinical reasoning/synthesis
   Rationale: The facts provided in the question indicate that the client has a condition in which the ability to continue to adapt is compromised. A treatment plan needs to be designed to support recovery without placing additional strain on the system. Since this question is asking for which of the possible answers is something that should not be done, then attempting to generate outcomes in ten sessions or less would seem to be contrary to the best treatment plan.

5. **a**
   Application and concept identification
   Rationale: The treatment plan approach of condition management is defined in the question. The correct answer would conform to this definition. Answer a is correct. Answers b and c are therapeutic change, and answer d may be a breach of scope of practice.

6. **b**
   Application and concept identification
   Rationale: The question presents data, and the answers are asking for a treatment approach in response to the data. Referral in this situation seems overly cautious since there is a reason for the discomfort and it fits the criteria of stage one, which is easily reversible. Reversible conditions respond to therapeutic change.

7. **c**
   Application and concept identification
   Rationale: Palliative care reduces suffering and would be most appropriate for the man with terminal cancer. This does not mean that the other three conditions would not respond to palliation, but condition management would be more appropriate.

8. **d**
   Factual recall
   Rationale: The correct answer defines health. The other three answers indicate that the mechanisms of health are breaking down.

9. **c**
   Factual recall
   Rationale: The correct answer defines pathology.

10. **d**
    Factual recall
    Rationale: This question type asks for the identification of terminology used in the correct context.

11. **b**
    Factual recall
    Rationale: The correct answer defines a sign in relation to the information presented in the question. Signs are objective and observable information. The wrong answers are all examples of subjective data.

12. **c**
    Factual recall
    Rationale: The correct answer is the definition of homeostasis.

13. **b**
    Factual recall
    Rationale: This is a terminology question. All the terms need to be defined to identify the correct answer.

14. **c**
    Factual recall
    Rationale: This is the type of question where some of the components are provided in the question and the last in the sequence needs to be identified.

15. **d**
    Factual recall
    Rationale: This is a terminology question. All the terms need to be defined to identify the correct answer.

16. **c**
Factual recall
Rationale: The question provides information about a benefit of massage in relation to good tissue healing, which involves promoting regulation and keeping replacement minimal.

17. **a**
Factual recall
Rationale: The question provides an outcome for a massage method and then asks for the best approach to achieve this goal.

18. **b**
Application and concept identification
Rationale: The question asks for the situation in which creating therapeutic inflammation would be appropriate. Answers a, c, and d are all contraindicated for this approach.

19. **c**
Factual recall
Rationale: The correct answer is the definition of chronic pain.

20. **c**
Factual recall
Rationale: All of the answers describe pain, but it is important to differentiate between types of pain to identity indications and contraindications for massage.

21. **d**
Factual recall
Rationale: The correct answer is the definition of somatic pain. All the terms need to be defined. Soma means body and is used to describe the soft tissue to include skin, muscles, joints, tendons, and fascia.

22. **b**
Factual recall
Rationale: The question presents another pain type—referred pain.

23. **d**
Factual recall
Rationale: It is very important to recognize the viscerally referred pain pattern to identify a need for referral. This question addresses this factual content.

24. **a**
Factual recall
Rationale: It is very important to recognize the viscerally referred pain pattern to identify a need for referral. This question addresses this factual content.

25. **c**
Application and concept identification
Rationale: The question addresses issues pertaining to treatment plans for different types of pain. Chronic and intractable pain are addressed with symptom relief. Chronic pain may be addressed with aggressive methods if the client has adaptive capacity. Answer c is the correct answer for acute pain, and answer d is misuse of terminology.

26. **d**
Factual recall
Rationale: Terms in the question need to be defined and the referred pain patterns of impingement of all the plexuses identified in order to identify the correct referred pain pattern, which would be into the head and neck area.

27. **a**
Factual recall
Rationale: Terms in the question need to be defined and the referred pain patterns of impingement of all the plexuses identified in order to identify the correct referred pain pattern, which would be into the leg and gluteal area without lumbar pain.

28. **b**
Application and concept identification
Rationale: First, impingement syndromes need to be defined. Then the proper method is chosen to address the condition. Since massage most specifically addresses soft tissue nerve entrapment by increasing the resting length of muscles, answer b is the best method of those listed.

29. **d**
Factual recall
Rationale: The correct answer is the definition of regional contraindication.

30. **c**
Factual recall
Rationale: Both benign and malignant need to be defined to choose the correct answer.

31. **c**
Factual recall
Rationale: The similarity between medication effect and massage benefit is seen in these three basic interactions—replace, stimulate, and inhibit.

32. **b**
    Factual recall
    Rationale: The terms need to be defined in relation to medication usage. When massage and medication both perform a similar function, it is a synergistic relationship.

33. **d**
    Application and concept identification
    Rationale: Various areas on the body are susceptible to pressure damage.

34. **c**
    Factual recall
    Rationale: The answer provides the definition of intractable pain.

35. **d**
    Factual recall
    Rationale: The question defines risk factors.

36. **c**
    Factual recall
    Rationale: The question defines signs.

37. **a**
    Factual recall
    Rationale: The question defines connective tissue.

38. **b**
    Application and concept identification
    Rationale: The action of the medication needs to be determined to identify which massage application would be detrimental in combination with the medication. This is an example of the many questions that can be written about medication and massage applications for safe practice. An anticoagulant is a blood thinner, so friction may cause bruising.

39. **a**
    Application and concept identification
    Rationale: This question asks about endangerment sites.

40. **c**
    Clinical reasoning/synthesis
    Rationale: Each of the possible answers needs to be an analyzed to determine what would be safe for massage and what needs more expert diagnosis. Answer a provides facts about edema, the severity of the condition, and a logical explanation. No referral would be necessary. Answer b does not represent a condition in relation to massage. Answer c is the correct answer since there is no explanation for the condition and bruising can be a sign of more serious pathology. Answer d does not represent a contraindication unless there is something contraindicated with the medication.

18

Hygiene, Sanitation, and Safety

Questions

1. Pathogenic disease-causing organisms include _____.

   a. Dirt, sweat, and grime
   b. Paint, tar, and dust
   c. Viruses, bacteria, and fungi
   d. Smoking, drinking, and washing

2. A group of simple parasitic organisms that are similar to plants but have no chlorophyll and live on skin or mucous membranes are _____.

   a. Viruses
   b. Fungi — *body's normal flora contains many fungi* *single cell org*
   c. Bacteria
   d. Protozoa → *infections*

3. Pathogens are spread by three main routes. Which of those below is one of these?

   a. Opportunistic invasion *pathogens transmitted blood or body fluid*
   b. Clean uniform
   c. Intact skin
   d. Aseptic technique

4. The three primary ways pathogens are spread are person-to-person contact, environmental contact, and _____.

   a. Handwashing
   b. Universal precautions
   c. Shoes
   d. Opportunistic invasion

5. Pressurized steam bath would be an example of what common aseptic technique?

   a. Isolation
   b. Sterilization
   c. Disinfections
   d. Universal precautions

6. The simplest, most effective deterrent to the spread of disease is _____.

   a. Handwashing
   b. Sterilization technique
   c. Using a towel barrier
   d. Keeping shots up-to-date

7. An example of disinfection is _____.

   a. Chemicals such as alcohol or soaps
   b. Extreme temperature
   c. Sanitary disposal of tissues
   d. Pressurized steam bath

8. You are running behind today and your next client has been waiting for 15 minutes. It is most important that you _____.

   a. Maintain your scheduled appointments on time
   b. Have materials and activities available for clients to entertain themselves
   c. Make sure sheets and linens are changed and equipment disinfected between massages
   d. Apologize to the client for being late

9. *Acquired immunodeficiency syndrome is defined as* _____.

    a. An inflammatory process caused by a virus

    b. Human immunodeficiency virus

    c. A group of clinical symptoms caused by a dysfunction in the body's immune system

    d. A disease contracted by casual contact such as shaking hands or sharing bathroom facilities

10. *Which of the following is **not** a safe professional practice?*

    a. Assisting the elderly on and off the massage table

    b. Burning candles for atmosphere in the massage room

    c. Maintaining good lighting in massage areas

    d. Regularly checking cables of portable massage tables

11. *Universal precautions are defined as* _____.

    a. Emergency care given to all ill or injured persons before medical help arrives

    b. Procedures developed by the CDC to prevent the spread of contagious disease

    c. The process by which all microorganisms are destroyed

    d. The process by which pathogens are destroyed

Answers and Discussion

1. **c**
   Factual recall
   Rationale: The correct answer provides examples of pathogenic organisms.

2. **b**
   Factual recall
   Rationale: The question defines fungi.

3. **a**
   Factual recall
   Rationale: This question is an example of how the same information can be tested in an exam question. See question 4. The three wrong answers are methods that prevent the spread of disease.

4. **d**
   Factual recall
   Rationale: This question is an example of how the same information can be tested in an exam question. See question 3. The three wrong answers are methods that prevent the spread of disease.

5. **b**
   Factual recall
   Rationale: The question provides an example of sterilization. All the terms need to be defined to identify the correct answer.

6. **a**
   Factual recall
   Rationale: Proper handwashing is essential to sanitary massage therapy practice.

7. **a**
   Factual recall
   Rationale: The correct answer is an example of disinfection.

8. **c**
   Clinical reasoning/synthesis
   Rationale: This type of question asks for a decision. The correct answer is the one that best conforms with standards of sanitary practice. All of the answers are correct, but safety of the client always is a priority.

9. **c**
   Factual recall
   Rationale: The correct answer is the definition of acquired immunodeficiency syndrome.

10. **b**
    Factual recall
    Rationale: The correct answer is the one containing incorrect information. Always read questions written in this style very carefully. An open flame is a safety hazard. All safety hazards need to be identified to promote safe professional practice.

11. **b**
    Factual recall
    Rationale: Universal precautions are a specific protocol of sanitary procedures developed by the Centers for Disease Control and Prevention.

19

Body Mechanics

Questions

1. When a practitioner is in a relaxed standing posture supporting the gravitational line with the normal knee-locked position, which muscles are used for balance?

   a. Psoas
   b. Gastrocnemius
   c. Hamstrings
   d. Quadriceps

2. What is the most efficient standing position?

   a. Symmetrical
   b. Wide stance (shoulder length apart)
   c. Asymmetrical
   d. Lead foot with the pressure on it

3. Most massage applications use a force generated _____.

   a. Downward
   b. Forward
   c. Downward and forward
   d. Forward and across

4. When one is applying compressive force down and forward, weight is most efficient if kept _____.

   a. On the back leg and foot
   b. On the front leg and knee
   c. On the back foot and toes
   d. On the front foot and toes

5. A massage professional is feeling strain in the shoulders and arms after doing four massage sessions. Which of the following is the most logical reason?

   a. The massage professional is using muscle strength in the arms to exert force
   b. The massage professional is standing in an asymmetrical stance
   c. The client is positioned for best mechanical advantage
   d. The massage professional is effectively leaning up hill

6. A massage practitioner has been experiencing increasingly severe low-back pain. The practice is full time with 20 clients per week. What could the massage practitioner do to reduce back strain?

   a. Bend the knees while performing massage
   b. Raise the table height to prevent torso bending
   c. Keep the head forward and down to change the center of gravity
   d. Externally rotate the back foot away from the line of force

7. A client keeps complaining of discomfort at the end of the massage stroke. What is happening?

   a. The practitioner is pushing with the legs
   b. The practitioner is off balance and using counterpressure
   c. The skin is being pulled from lack of lubricant
   d. The compressive force is distributed over a narrow base at the end of the stroke

8. A massage professional is complaining of pain in the wrist and near the elbow. Which of the following is an appropriate corrective action?

    a. Maintain the hands in a clenched fist to promote stability
    b. Increase the movement of the stroke at the shoulder joint
    c. Relax the hand and fingers during massage
    d. Shift the compressive force to the fingers and thumb

9. Observation of a fellow massage practitioner indicates that the shoulder girdle is aligned with the pelvic girdle, the pressure-bearing arm opposite the weight-bearing leg, the fingers relaxed, the head up, the back straight, the elbows bent, and the stance asymmetrical. Which of these areas needs correction?

    a. Elbows
    b. Stance
    c. Back position
    d. Shoulder position

10. A massage professional is feeling strain in the knees. Which of the following is the most logical cause?

    a. Doing massage on hard floors
    b. Working with clients in the side-lying position
    c. Keeping the knees flexed and static
    d. Moving whenever the arm reach is beyond 60 degrees

11. Increasing levels of pressure are achieved by _____.

    a. Moving closer to the massage table
    b. Moving away from the massage table
    c. Standing on the toes
    d. Shifting the weight-bearing foot to the front

12. When stretching the legs of a client by applying a pull against the ankle, the massage practitioner should _____.

    a. Fix the feet and pull with the shoulders
    b. Move to a symmetrical stance and lean back
    c. Maintain asymmetrical stance, lean back, keeping the back straight
    d. Bend the knees and push back

Answers and Discussion

1. **b**
   Factual recall
   Rationale: The relaxed standing position conserves muscle energy, while maintaining balance with the gastrocnemius and soleus muscles.

2. **c**
   Factual recall
   Rationale: The incorrect answers are all fatiguing.

3. **c**
   Factual recall
   Rationale: Two directional forces are used with massage—compressive force down with a forward momentum.

4. **a**
   Factual recall
   Rationale: This question is an example of how information presented in either the question or the possible answers can relate to other questions in the examination. This question relates to question 3. A person who did not know the answer to question 3 would find it in question 4 by the way it is worded. In this question the correct answer describes proper weight distribution.

5. **a**
   Clinical reasoning/synthesis
   Rationale: Facts in the question suggest that something is incorrect with the delivery of the massage. The answers need to be analyzed against the question to make the decision about the cause. The incorrect answers describe appropriate body mechanics, while the correct answer is a logical explanation for the strain in the arms and shoulders.

6. **b**
   Clinical reasoning/synthesis
   Rationale: The facts in the question are: low-back pain that is getting worse and full-time massage practice. The possible answers need to be analyzed for the logical reason for this condition and what could be done to correct the problem. Answer a would likely make the condition worse and add knee strain. Answer b is the correct answer. Both answers c and d are actions that would increase the strain.

7. **d**
   Application and concept identification
   Rationale: If the massage practitioner shifts the weight to the front foot at the end of the stroke, the focus of the pressure is smaller and would be uncomfortable.

8. **c**
   Clinical reasoning/synthesis
   Rationale: The question indicates that something is wrong with the body mechanics, resulting in pain. All three of the incorrect answers would increase the pain.

9. **a**
   Application and concept identification
   Rationale: The question provides information about correct body mechanics except one area, bent elbows.

10. **c**
    Clinical reasoning/synthesis
    Rationale: The question asks for a decision on the cause of knee pain. After analysis of each answer, the only one that is logical is flexed and static knees.

11. **b**
    Factual recall
    Rationale: The center of gravity changes, resulting in increased pressure if the weight-bearing foot is moved further away from the table, but not to the point that one stands on the toes.

12. **c**
    Application and concept identification
    Rationale: This massage outcome would be accomplished most efficiently by using the method described in the correct answer.

20

Preparation for Massage

Questions

1. *The most important stability feature of a portable massage table is _____.*

   a. Frame
   b. Cable support
   c. Adjustable legs
   d. Center hinge

2. *A client is particularly concerned with safely and is afraid of falling. Of the following massage equipment, which would make the client most comfortable?*

   a. Mat
   b. Stationary table
   c. Portable table
   d. Chair

3. *Regardless of the type of draping material used, which of the following is required?*

   a. Disposable
   b. Large
   c. Opaque
   d. Cotton fabric

4. *To maintain sanitary practice, draping material must be _____.*

   a. Laundered in hot soapy water with a disinfectant such as bleach
   b. Sterilized and heat pressed
   c. Professionally laundered
   d. Warm, large enough to cover the client, and different colors

5. *To prevent allergic reactions, all lubricant should be _____.*

   a. Oil based
   b. Water based
   c. Dispensed in sanitary fashion
   d. Scent free

6. *The purpose of lubricant is _____.*

   a. To moisturize the skin
   b. To reduce friction on the skin
   c. To transport nutrients
   d. Counterirritation

7. *A massage professional has just rented office space and fully decorated the area. There is a window in the massage room and both overhead and indirect lighting. There is a central thermostat in another area, but the massage room has both a fan and an electric heater to adjust temperature. The small waiting area is bright and comfortable, with many sorts of flowering plants. There is a private restroom just off the waiting room. The massage room does not have a closet but does have hooks for the clients' clothing. A closed cabinet holds supplies. The business area is small but has a locked file cabinet and small desk. What suggestion would you make for improving the massage environment?*

   a. Add an aromatherapy atomizer
   b. Put a lock on the massage room door
   c. Move the file cabinet into the massage room
   d. Remove the flowering plants

8. *Which environment is the most difficult for maintaining professional boundaries?*

   a. Public events
   b. Private office commercial building
   c. On-site residence
   d. Home office

9. *A massage practitioner has been seeing the same client weekly for 3 months. The client often discusses personal issues with the massage practitioner. Last session the massage professional provided some reading information to help the client and talked with the client about how the practitioner had dealt with a similar issue. The client has canceled the last two appointments. What is the most logical cause?*

   a. Feedback about the massage broke down
   b. Conversation with the client overshadowed the massage session
   c. Gender issues are influencing the session
   d. The orientation process needs to be repeated

10. *A massage professional is preparing an orientation process for a new client. The professional has developed the following checklist: Show client massage area, where to change and hang clothes, massage table draping and positioning, how to get on and off the massage table, music choices, and restrooms. Explain charts and equipment, lubricant types, sanitary procedures, and privacy methods. What did the massage professional forget?*

    a. To explain the general idea of massage flow
    b. To provide a centering meditation with the client
    c. To provide education on self-help
    d. To introduce the client to products for sale

11. *A client complains of a mild general low back pain. Which of the following is appropriate?*

    a. Use side-lying position with knee support
    b. Work with client prone, using support under the ankles
    c. Work with client supine, using support only under the neck
    d. Position client in seated position and avoid supports

12. *A client is quite shy and modest. Which of the following draping methods would be the best choice?*

    a. Contoured draping with towels
    b. Partial body towel draping
    c. Full body sheet and towel draping
    d. Sheet draping with no towels

13. *In which situation would you stay in the massage room and assist a client on and off the massage table?*

    a. A client in the first trimester of pregnancy
    b. A 65-year-old male with diabetes
    c. An elderly female with high blood pressure
    d. An adolescent with a wrist cast

14. *An adolescent athlete is coming for massage with a parent. You have been informed that the client is uncomfortable with disrobing. Which of the following is the most logical alternative?*

    a. An educational session
    b. A draping demonstration
    c. Working only with the feet
    d. Having the client wear loose shorts and T-shirt

15. *A client regularly lingers after the massage session to talk. The massage professional gets behind schedule because of this. What is the most likely cause of this problem?*

    a. Policies regarding leaving promptly after the massage were not addressed and reinforced
    b. The client requires a longer appointment
    c. The client needs more frequent appointments
    d. The massage professional is displaying transference

Answers and Discussion

1. **b**
   Factual recall
   Rationale: The cable support is the structural design component for stability, and the center hinge is the weak point.

2. **a**
   Application and concept identification
   Rationale: The mat would allow work to be done on the floor, where falling would not be an issue.

3. **c**
   Factual recall
   Rationale: Draping material provides warmth and modesty, so the material must be opaque.

4. **a**
   Factual recall
   Rationale: Sanitation is a priority, using disinfection appropriate for linens.

5. **d**
   Factual recall
   Rationale: The most common reason for allergic reaction to a lubricant is the volatile oils that are used to scent the product.

6. **b**
   Factual recall
   Rationale: The only reason for lubricant is to reduce skin friction when doing gliding or kneading massage methods. All other reasons, such as medicinal or cosmetic ones, may be a breach in the scope of practice.

7. **d**
   Clinical reasoning/synthesis
   Rationale: All of the recommendations and cautions for creating a massage environment need to be reviewed to decide what needs to be changed in the massage area described by the question. Answer a is not recommended, since scents may cause allergic reactions in sensitive individuals and personal preference varies. A lock on the massage door can be considered entrapment, so it is inappropriate. Since the file cabinet is locked, confidentiality is maintained. It is recommended to remove the plants, again since many people are allergic to them.

8. **c**
   Factual recall
   Rationale: Of the four answers provided, going to a client's home presents the most difficult boundary issues.

9. **b**
   Clinical reasoning/synthesis
   Rationale: A summary of the facts provided in the question indicates that boundary issues have been breached and conversation with the client was inappropriate. To identify the correct answer, one must understand the concepts of feedback, gender issues, and an appropriate orientation process.

10. **a**
    Application and concept identification
    Rationale: The question reflects a comprehensive, first-client orientation process. It is important to explain the massage flow to clients so that they are more comfortable with the process. The incorrect answers either describe a boundary violation or are not part of the orientation process.

11. **a**
    Application and concept identification
    Rationale: Prone and supine positioning tend to aggravate low back pain. Even a seated position can be tiring to the low back. Therefore the side-lying position is the best choice.

12. **c**
    Clinical reasoning/synthesis
    Rationale: The question presents a common massage practice situation. In this situation the wrong answers do not provide enough body coverage to accommodate this client.

13. **c**
    Application and concept identification
    Rationale: When safety is a concern, the client should be assisted on and off the table. When considering the client conditions presented, the elderly female with blood pressure concerns is correct because she could be dizzy after the massage.

14. **d**
    Clinical reasoning/synthesis
    Rationale: Massage can be done without the client removing clothing. Methods can be modified to adjust to the situation or the client can wear clothing that is easy to work around. It is not necessary to change the client's beliefs with a demonstration of draping or an educational session when having the client wear shorts and loose shirt solves the problem.

15. **a**
    Clinical reasoning/synthesis
    Rationale: As with all of these types of questions, there is a decision about what to do in a particular situation or what is wrong or right with the situation presented in the question. In this question, a client does not leave after the session, which makes it difficult for the professional to maintain a work schedule. Usually this is because the policies and client rules were not enforced from the beginning, as described in the correct answer. Wrong answers b and c would predispose to future problems, and answer d is an incorrect word usage.

21

Massage Manipulations and Techniques

Questions

1. Massage manipulations are _____.

   a. Skillful use of the hands and forearms to directly affect the soft tissue
   b. Skillful use of the hands to directly affect the joints
   c. Application of methods using heat and equipment to affect soft tissue
   d. Application of compressive forces to affect meridians

2. A massage practitioner uses massage manipulations in a brisk and specific way. Which of the following client goals is best served by this approach?

   a. Decreased alertness
   b. Increased parasympathetic response
   c. Decreased sensory awareness
   d. Increased alertness

3. A client has an outcome goal for the massage of increased circulation and range of motion for the knee. Which of the following is the best approach?

   a. Reflexive methods focused on chemical changes
   b. Mechanical methods focused on the area
   c. Mechanical methods to reflexively influence neuroactivity
   d. Reflexive methods to increase compressive force to the viscera

4. A massage client is unhappy with the massage. The main complaint is a feeling of choppiness and lack of continuity. Which of the following qualities of touch is most responsible?

   a. Depth of pressure
   b. Drag
   c. Rhythm
   d. Direction

5. Which of the following methods is most beneficial for abdominal massage to mechanically encourage fecal movement in the large intestine?

   a. Effleurage
   b. Resting position
   c. Tapotement
   d. Compression

6. Which of the following methods has as its primary effect a lifting of the tissue away from underlying structures?

   a. Compression
   b. Petrissage
   c. Gliding
   d. Vibration

Answers are on pages 153–154.

7. *A client reports a sensitivity to lubricant during the history and would like a massage in which no lubricant is used. Which method would be* **inappropriate?**

   a. Shaking
   b. Compression
   c. Kneading
   d. Effleurage

8. *When the outcome for the massage is to produce parasympathetic dominance, which combination of methods would be the best choice?*

   a. Gliding, rocking, and passive joint movement
   b. Compression, shaking, and friction
   c. Active joint movement, reciprocal inhibition, and rocking
   d. Tapotement, compression, and vibration

9. *A client complains of restricted range of motion in the shoulder. The primary outcome for the massage is to increase shoulder mobility. Which method would be the best choice?*

   a. Friction
   b. Muscle energy
   c. Hydrotherapy
   d. Resting stroke

10. *A client requests that tapotement be used at the end of the massage to stimulate the nervous system. Which is the best choice for the face?*

    a. Hacking
    b. Cupping
    c. Tapping
    d. Slapping

11. *Which of the following methods would be best for assessing for the physiologic and pathologic motion barrier?*

    a. Passive joint movement
    b. Active resistive movement
    c. Postisometric relaxation
    d. Concentric isotonic contraction

12. *Which of the following is produced voluntarily?*

    a. Joint play
    b. Arthrokinematic movement
    c. Osteokinematic movement
    d. Joint end-feel

13. *Which component is essential for effective application of joint movement?*

    a. Stabilization to isolate the movement to the targeted joint
    b. Tapotement to stimulate the joint kinesthetic receptors
    c. High-velocity manipulative movement
    d. Cross-directional tissue stretching to cause traction on the joint capsule

14. *A client's muscles cramp when the massage professional attempts to use postisometric relaxation to lengthen a shortened group of muscles. Which of the following methods would be a better choice to lengthen the muscle group?*

    a. Skin rolling
    b. Active resistive joint movement
    c. Reciprocal inhibition
    d. Stretching

15. *A client is feeling fatigued and does not wish to participate during the massage. Instead the client wishes to remain passive and quiet. Which of the following muscle energy methods would be appropriate?*

    a. Positional release
    b. Pulsed muscle energy
    c. Integrated approach
    d. Approximation

16. *Which method is being described? Isolate the target muscle in passive contraction. Have the client contract the antagonist group. Have the client relax and then lengthen the target muscles.*

    a. Postisometric relaxation
    b. Reciprocal inhibition
    c. Contract-relax antagonist contract
    d. Pulsed muscle energy

17. *A client has been receiving massage weekly for 2 months. The main goal for the massage is increased mobility in the lumbar and hip region. The client has experienced stiffness and reduced ability since a fall off a bike 2 years ago. General massage and muscle energy methods with lengthening have produced mild improvement. Which of the following mechanical methods has the potential to increase results?*

    a. Lymphatic drainage
    b. Stretching
    c. Contract/relax
    d. Strain-counterstrain

18. *A client is ticklish, particularly on the chest. Which method would be the best choice to use in this area?*

    a. Compression over the client's own hand
    b. Friction
    c. Gentle effleurage
    d. Fingertip compression

19. *A client is requesting extensive massage to the neck and upper shoulders. Which is the most efficient client position to easily massage these areas?*

    a. Prone
    b. Supine
    c. Seated
    d. Side-lying

20. *Which method is beneficial to use on the hands and feet to stimulate lymphatic movement?*

    a. Superficial effleurage
    b. Skin rolling
    c. Vibration
    d. Pumping compression

21. *A client complains of a stiff and stuck feeling in the lumbar area. Assessment indicates that the fascia in that area is thick and adhered to the underlying tissue. Which method would best restore pliability to this tissue?*

    a. Skin rolling
    b. Shaking
    c. Friction
    d. Vibration

22. *A client has a lot of body hair on his back. During the first massage lubricant was used. At the return visit the client requests that lubricant not be used on his body where there are large amounts of hair. Which method could be used?*

    a. Gliding
    b. Kneading
    c. Compression
    d. Petrissage

23. *A major contraindication to massage of the legs is _____.*

    a. Acne
    b. Brachial nerve compression
    c. Disk compression
    d. Thrombophlebitis

24. *A client likes to have the back massaged and asks that most of the massage time be focused on the back. The client continues to complain that the massage is not very effective in reducing back pain. What explanation can be given to the client?*

    a. The soft tissue of the back often is tight because of extensive pulling and shortening of the tissues in the chest; massage of the chest may help
    b. Massage to the back limits blood flow, so the soft tissues remain in contracture
    c. Massage on the extremities would be better to reduce the pain in this area since the mechanical effect is more concentrated
    d. The connective tissues of the back respond best to reflexive measures, and using a more generalized approach would provide relief

25. *Which of the following methods is best for general broad applications when lubricant is requested?*

    a. Petrissage
    b. Compression
    c. Effleurage
    d. Vibration

Answers are on pages 153–154.

26. Which of the following is of most concern when massaging the face?

    a. Proximity to mucous membranes and transmission of pathogens
    b. The skin of the face is thin
    c. Facial muscles are weak
    d. Compression damages underlying cranial sutures

27. A client is complaining about pain and stiffness in the neck but is particularly sensitive to pressure used in the neck area, flinching and stiffening in a protective stance whenever the neck is massaged. The current approach is to primarily use petrissage with the client in the prone position. What is the best alternative?

    a. Change position to supine and use effleurage
    b. Use side-lying position and broad-based compression
    c. Combine passive range of motion, muscle energy, and friction with client seated
    d. Have client seated and then use deep petrissage

28. Which of the following body areas requires special attention to draping?

    a. Hand
    b. Leg
    c. Chest
    d. Shoulder

29. Which of the following body areas is often massaged longer than is effective?

    a. Hands
    b. Abdomen
    c. Legs
    d. Back

30. A client arrives late for a massage appointment. The remaining time is 30 minutes. The goal for the session is general relaxation. Which combination is the best choice to achieve desired outcomes in the allotted time?

    a. Back, gluteals, and hips
    b. Face, hands, and feet
    c. Hands, arms, and back
    d. Face, neck, and shoulders

Answers and Discussion

1. **a**
Factual recall
Rationale: The correct answer is the definition of massage manipulations.

2. **d**
Application and concept identification
Rationale: This type of massage application would stimulate the body, increasing alertness.

3. **b**
Clinical reasoning/synthesis
Rationale: Both goals of circulation enhancement and increased range of motion are achieved though mechanical methods. Analysis of the incorrect answers indicates that the information is either flawed or not in context with the question.

4. **c**
Application and concept identification
Rationale: To answer the question all the terms need to be defined and then compared to the data in the question. The rhythm of the massage was not appropriate to the client's needs.

5. **a**
Application and concept identification
Rationale: The question asks for the best methods to achieve an outcome in a specific body area or function. This question is representative of the many types of questions that can be developed around this content. To answer the question, the application and physiologic effect of all the massage methods need to be understood. In this particular question, effleurage is the best choice.

6. **b**
Factual recall
Rationale: The question defines petrissage. All the terms need to be defined to answer the question.

7. **d**
Factual recall
Rationale: Only effleurage requires the use of lubricant.

8. **a**
Application and concept identification
Rationale: To answer this question all the terms need to be defined and the physiologic outcome determined. Only the correct answer lists those methods that do not stimulate a sympathetic response.

9. **b**
Clinical reasoning/synthesis
Rationale: Each method needs to be evaluated for effectiveness in relation to the goal stated in the question. All of the methods listed may provide benefit, but muscle energy methods are most specifically used to increase range of motion by creating a more normal muscle resting length.

10. **c**
Application and concept identification
Rationale: Each term needs to be defined and its application described. Only tapping is appropriate for the face.

11. **a**
Application and concept identification
Rationale: Each term needs to be defined and its use for assessment described. Also the terms in the question need to be understood to interpret the question. Passive joint movement is the best choice for assessment of range of motion, since all the others involve a muscle contraction.

12. **c**
Factual recall
Rationale: This information was also covered in the science study, and the overlap of information is apparent. The terms need to be defined to identify osteokinematic movement as the correct answer.

13. **a**
Application and concept identification
Rationale: Only if proper stabilization is used can joint movement isolate its effects.

14. **c**
Application and concept identification
Rationale: All the terms need to be defined to understand that postisometric relaxation methods first have the target muscle contract. In this instance the contraction is causing cramping. Reciprocal inhibition would make use of the antagonist contracting, bypassing the tendency to cramp.

15. **d**
Factual recall
Rationale: After the terminology and application of the methods are defined, only approximation uses direct application by the massage professional to affect the receptors and does not require that the client actively contract muscle groups.

16. **b**
Factual recall
Rationale: The question describes reciprocal inhibition. To answer the question, one must understand how to apply the other muscle energy methods listed.

17. **b**
Clinical reasoning/synthesis
Rationale: First the question needs to be analyzed to identify the reasons for the client's symptoms. The question describes reflexive methods and indicates that there has been a small improvement. The question asks for the mechanical application that would improve results based on the goal. Lymphatic drainage is not focused on the goal. Answer b is correct since stretching mechanically affects the connective tissue. Answers c and d are other types of muscle energy methods. This question is an example of the hundreds of questions that can be written to test this type of content.

18. **a**
Factual recall
Rationale: The incorrect answers may increase the tickle sensation.

19. **d**
Application and concept identification
Rationale: Any of the possible answers would allow the neck to be massaged, but the side-lying position provides the best mechanical advantage for the massage therapist to use body mechanics.

20. **d**
Application and concept identification
Rationale: Compression on the lymphatic plexuses located in the hands and feet would provide the best outcome of the methods listed as possible answers.

21. **a**
Application and concept identification
Rationale: Skin rolling is the best method of those listed to affect the connective tissue.

22. **c**
Application and concept identification
Rationale: Compression does not require lubricant.

23. **d**
Factual recall
Rationale: The veins in the legs are more susceptible to blood clot development.

24. **a**
Clinical reasoning/synthesis
Rationale: Each of the possible answers needs to be analyzed to understand it in relation to the question posed. The wrong answers in this question present misinformation. Requesting massage focused on the back is a common occurrence in massage. Usually back tension is caused by shortening of the soft tissue structures of the chest.

25. **c**
Factual recall
Rationale: The question describes a common application of effleurage.

26. **a**
Factual recall
Rationale: Pathogen transmission through the mucous membranes in the face is a concern. The delicate nature of the facial structures is less of a concern.

27. **b**
Clinical reasoning/synthesis
Rationale: The key to the correct answer is sensitivity to pressure. Only the correct answer provides a method that can be applied lightly, while the side-lying position allows the client to see more of what is happening, making the client more comfortable.

28. **c**
Factual recall
Rationale: The chest area should be carefully draped because of breast tissue.

29. **d**
Factual recall
Rationale: This content was addressed in a previous question and is an example of how content often appears in different forms in an examination. This can be helpful since the different wording may trigger the correct answer in a question that posed difficulties in some other area of the exam.

30. **b**
Clinical reasoning/synthesis
Rationale: The problem presented by the question is which body areas to massage in a limited time to achieve the strongest relaxation effect. Each combination needs to be reviewed to assess for physiologic effects when massage is applied. Face, hands, and feet have the largest nervous system distribution.

22

Assessment Procedures for Developing a Care Plan

Questions

1. *A massage practitioner identifies an area of restricted tissue and immediately uses skin rolling to increase connective tissue pliability. How did this interfere with assessment processes?*

   a. The localized treatment did not prove effective
   b. The pattern was changed before it was understood
   c. The therapist did not chart the area prior to the massage
   d. The method was not appropriate to the condition

2. *A client seems nervous and unwilling to provide information during the history-taking process. The massage therapist is becoming impatient. What is lacking?*

   a. Rapport between client and practitioner
   b. Prior information from the physician
   c. State-dependent memory status
   d. Proper clinical reasoning skills

3. *When are data collected during the assessment process interpreted as to patterns of dysfunction and methods of massage application?*

   a. As the history taking progresses
   b. During the physical assessment
   c. As the information is charted in the subjective section
   d. After the data have been collected and analyzed

4. *During the initial greeting, a client seems generally healthy and in good spirits; however, when the client is speaking the breathing pattern seems strained. What assessment process is being used?*

   a. Palpation
   b. Physical assessment
   c. Interviewing
   d. Observation

5. *A massage practitioner asks a client the following question, "Please explain to me how you would like to feel after the massage." What is correct about this communication?*

   a. The massage practitioner used an open-ended question
   b. The massage practitioner directed the response to reduce rapport
   c. The practitioner was formulating a response during listening to the answer
   d. A closed-ended interview was used to effectively use time

6. *A massage practitioner carefully listens to a client during the interview portion of the assessment process and then proceeds to the physical assessment. What communication step was forgotten?*

   a. Open-ended questions and analysis
   b. Charting and treatment plan development
   c. Summarizing and restating information
   d. Using understandable language

7. *A vacationing client will only have one massage from the massage practitioner. Which is the appropriate assessment process?*

   a. Subjective history taking for possible referral combined with a physical assessment for symmetry and gait assessment for optimal movement patterns

   b. Palpation assessment of soft tissues to identify treatment areas

   c. Subjective and objective assessment for contraindications

   d. Interviewing for client's quantitative goals

8. *During postural assessment the massage professional observes that the client's shoulder girdle is rotated to the left. Which of the following histories is most likely to be the cause?*

   a. The client regularly reaches to the left when answering the phone

   b. The client often wears boots when riding horses

   c. The client does weight-bearing exercise with machines three times a week

   d. The client wears tight clothing

9. *A regular client has a grade 2 left ankle sprain and is using a crutch to maintain balance when walking. During assessment of posture, the massage therapist notices an elevated right shoulder. What is happening to cause this?*

   a. The client is closing an open kinetic chain pattern

   b. The muscles of the right lower leg are inhibited

   c. The symmetrical stance is enhanced

   d. The body is displaying compensation patterns

10. *When one is observing for symmetry, which of the following is correct?*

   a. The shoulders should evenly roll forward, leveling the clavicles

   b. The circumference of the muscle mass in the legs should be similar

   c. The ribs should be fixed more on the left and springy on the right

   d. The patella should be pointed more medially

11. *Which of the following is part of a normal gait pattern?*

   a. The arms swing freely opposite the leg swing

   b. The knee is maintained in the "screw-home" mechanism

   c. The toes contact the floor first and then roll to the heel

   d. During push-off the foot is dorsiflexed

12. *While observing a client walk, the massage professional notices that the pelvis does not move evenly. The client complains of focused pain in the right sacral area. Which of the following is most correct?*

   a. Create a massage treatment plan describing specific treatment for sacroiliac dysfunction

   b. This information combined with other data may indicate the need for referral, with current massage focused on general nonspecific approaches

   c. Design a massage to lengthen the left leg to balance the pelvic rotation

   d. Immediately refer the client to a chiropractor for sacroiliac dysfunction

13. *During the massage the massage professional notices a temperature difference in the tissue of the lumbar area. One area the size of a quarter is warmer than the surrounding area. Which type of assessment is being used?*

   a. Postural assessment

   b. Gait assessment

   c. Palpation

   d. Muscle testing

14. *Which of the following is the most effective way to assess for potential areas of muscle hyperactivity when the focus of the palpation is on the surface of the skin?*

   a. Compressing until the striations of the underlying muscles are felt

   b. Light fingertip stroking to assess for areas of dampness or drag

   c. Skin rolling to assess for any adherence of superficial fascia to the skin

   d. Moving the skin on top of the superficial fascia to locate areas of bind

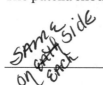

15. *When one is using passive joint movement as an assessment method, which of the following is being identified?*

    a) End feel
    b. Viscosity
    c. Vessels
    d. Pilomotor reflex

16. *Bilateral assessment of the dorsalis pedis pulse would provide information about _____.*

    a. Respiration
    b. Abdominal viscera
    c. Lymph nodes
    d. Arterial circulation

17. *During palpation assessment, the massage practitioner wishes to assess for the status of the acupuncture meridians. Where would the practitioner focus the assessment?*

    a. Tendons at the proximal attachment
    b. Ligament of synovial joints
    c. Grooves in fascial sheaths
    d. Myotomes

18. *Which of the following is **incorrect** when using strength muscle testing?*

    a. Isolate muscles and position attachments as close together as is comfortable
    b. Use a force sufficient to recruit a full response of the tested muscles and the surrounding muscles
    c. Use a slow and even counterpressure to pull or push the muscle out of the isolated position
    d. Compare muscle tests bilaterally for symmetry

19. *A client is complaining of weakness and heaviness in the muscles that flex the left thigh. During muscle testing, the muscle group is found to be inhibited. Based on gait patterns, which of the following muscle groups should also be inhibited?*

    a. Right arm flexors
    b. Left arm flexors
    c. Right thigh flexors
    d. Left thigh extensors

20. *During strength muscle testing, both the flexors and the extensors of the elbow seem equally strong. Why is this a dysfunctional pattern?*

    a. Gait patterns should inhibit the flexors
    b. Flexors should be about 25% stronger than extensors
    c. Extensors should be 30% stronger than adductors
    d. Postural muscles are inhibited by gait reflexes

21. *A client is experiencing spasms in the left thigh flexor muscles. An attempt to muscle test the area could result in a cramp. The massage professional remembers that activation of the gait reflexes can either facilitate or inhibit muscle contraction. Which group of muscles would the massage professional have the client contract in order to inhibit the left thigh flexors?*

    a. Left arm flexors
    b. Right arm flexors
    c. Left arm extensors
    d. Right thigh extensors

22. *If the area between C-7 and T-12 is pulled forward, making the chest concave, with a right rotation pattern making the right shoulder more forward than the left, where are the shortened soft tissues?*

    a. Anterior thorax on the right
    b. Right lumbar posterior
    c. Left thorax posterior
    d. Lower abdominal on the right

23. *During the interview process, a client continues to grab the tissue at the back of the neck and pull it. What is the most logical explanation for this gesture?*

    a. Nerve entrapment
    b. Joint compression
    c. Trigger point
    d. Connective tissue shortening

24. *A client has increased internal rotation of the right shoulder. Which of the following is the best massage approach to reverse the condition?*

   a. Frictioning and traction to the external rotators

   b. Muscle energy with lengthening and then stretching of the internal rotators

   c. Compression and tapotement to the internal rotators

   d. Stretching of the flexors and extensors with lengthening to the external rotators

25. *A physician refers a client for massage for circulation enhancement to the limbs. The client complains of cold hands and feet. Assessment indicates decreased pliability of the tissues around the elbows and knees. Work-related activities require repetitive movement in these areas. The massage professional presents three main approaches for the physician to consider:*

   1. *General massage and rest*
   2. *General massage with connective tissue stretching in the restricted areas*
   3. *Compression focused specifically to the arteries to encourage circulation*

   After considering all three options, the physician eliminates number 1 as too time consuming. Option 2 seems viable, but the client does not respond well to methods that may be painful. Option 3 seems too limited an approach to the massage professional. The decision is to begin with option 3 and expand to connective tissue methods when the client is able to tolerate them. Which part of this process best reflects brainstorming possibilities?

   a. Data collection

   b. Eliminations of options based on pros and cons

   c. Generating the options

   d. Assessment for more facts

26. *A client experienced an episode of severe low back pain 3 years ago. The diagnosis was a compressed disk at L-4. The condition has stabilized and pain is experienced only occasionally. Assessment indicates shortened lumbar fascia, increased lateral flexion to the right, and a high shoulder on the right. The massage professional specifically addressed these areas and noted improvement following the massage. The next day the client called complaining that the low back was in spasm. What is the most logical reason for what happened?*

   a. The phasic muscles were too weak to maintain posture

   b. The gait shifted so that there was a more normal heel strike

   c. Facilitated segments in the skeletal muscles went into spasm

   d. Resourceful compensation patterns were disturbed

27. *An objective measurement of connective tissue shortening in the lumbar area would be _____.*

   a. Measuring a skin fold by lifting the tissue

   b. Placing the client in the prone position and having her lift her chest off the table into extension

   c. Measurements of hot and cold skin temperature

   d. Palpation of adjacent pulse points for evenness

28. *When one is evaluating a treatment plan for successful client compliance, which of the following would provide the best information?*

   a. Any referral information from the heath care provider

   b. Completing a comprehensive physical assessment

   c. Generating multiple treatment options

   d. Indications of enthusiasm for the plan by the client and any support system

Answers and Discussion

1. **b**
   Application and concept identification
   Rationale: Assessment seeks to understand the reason for how the body is responding. The immediate application of an intervention method changed the condition before there was a chance to gather more information to understand the rest of the pattern.

2. **a**
   Factual recall
   Rationale: The question is providing an example of a breakdown in rapport.

3. **d**
   Factual recall
   Rationale: The sequence of assessment places interpretation of the data after data collection.

4. **d**
   Factual recall
   Rationale: The question provides an example of assessment by observation.

5. **a**
   Factual recall
   Rationale: The question provides an example of an open-ended question.

6. **c**
   Factual recall
   Rationale: The information received during the subjective assessment needs to be confirmed with the client to make sure it is understood.

7. **c**
   Factual recall
   Rationale: Single-session massage applications do not require an extensive assessment process but do need to identify possible contraindications.

8. **a**
   Clinical reasoning/synthesis
   Rationale: This is an example of a question that is asking for cause and effect. The effect is presented in the question, and the correct answer would present a logical explanation for the condition. The correct answer describes a repetitive movement pattern that, over time, could affect shoulder girdle position.

9. **d**
   Clinical reasoning/synthesis
   Rationale: This is an example of a question that is asking for cause and effect. The effect is presented in the question, and the correct answer would present a logical explanation for the condition. The correct answer is describes a common compensation pattern.

10. **b**
    Factual recall
    Rationale: Symmetry means the same on both sides, as reflected in the correct answer.

11. **a**
    Factual recall
    Rationale: Knowledge about a normal gait pattern is necessary to answer this question.

12. **b**
    Clinical reasoning/synthesis
    Rationale: The question provides symptoms that need to be correlated with the data in the correct answer. Answers a and d diagnose instead of assess the problem, which is outside the scope of practice for massage. There is no indication of leg imbalance. Through this elimination process, answer b emerges as the correct answer.

13. **c**
    Factual recall
    Rationale: The question gives an example of palpation.

14. **b**
    Factual recall
    Rationale: The only answer that focuses the palpation to the skin surface as explained in the question is answer b.

15. **a**
    Factual recall
    Rationale: End feel of joints would be the only logical answer.

16. **d**
    Factual recall
    Rationale: The terms need to be defined to correlate the data from the question with the correct answer, pulses assess arterial circulation.

17. **c**
    Factual recall
    Rationale: This question addresses both assessment and traditional Chinese medicine theory.

18. **b**
Application and concept identification
Rationale: The question asks for the wrong information, so three of the answers are accurate information. Do not let this be confusing. It is necessary to understand muscle-testing procedures to answer the question. Synergistic or fixator muscles should not be recruited. If this happens, the pressure is excessive.

19. **a**
Clinical reasoning/synthesis
Rationale: Normal gait pattern would determine a counterbalancing effect of the opposite arm and leg. If one group is inhibited, it is likely that the paired group is also inhibited.

20. **b**
Factual recall
Rationale: Flexors are typically stronger than extensors.

21. **a**
Clinical reasoning/synthesis
Rationale: The question is asking for a decision based on reflex patterns. The information about interactions of muscle groups during walking is necessary to answer the question. The counter-balancing arm swing during gait facilitates left arm and right leg muscles and right arm and left leg muscles whether the action is flexion or extension. If the leg is flexed, the opposite-arm flexors are also activated. If the leg is extended, then the extensors of the paired arm are also activated. Based on these interactions and on reciprocal inhibition of the antagonist group, the activated agonist is inhibited. To inhibit the left thigh flexor muscle groups, the client should contract the same-side left arm flexors. Many questions can be written using this basic information about muscle group interactions.

22. **a**
Clinical reasoning/synthesis
Rationale: The question asks for the causal factor when symptoms are present. Also necessary for these types of question is a strong anatomy and physiology base. The area described is the thorax. The facts of the question report the dysfunction as a pulling, which is typically contracted muscles or shortened connective tissue and often both. The shortened tissues described in the wrong answers would not result in the postural change.

23. **d**
Application and concept identification
Rationale: The client is gesturing. Pulling on tissue usually indicates connective tissue shortening.

24. **b**
Clinical reasoning/synthesis
Rationale: The facts state that assessment has identified an internal rotation of the right shoulder. To answer the question, one must know information about muscle and joint function and the physiologic effect of various massage methods. If internal rotation is increased, either the muscles that produce this movement are overly tense with inhibited external rotators or the connective tissue of the area is shortened, pulling the shoulder into internal rotation. If the condition is recent, it is probably neuromuscular; if it is chronic, there will likely be a myofascial shortening aspect to the dysfunction. Local intervention to the area is best achieved by combining muscle-energy methods to restore a normal resting length and stretching to increase pliability of the connective tissue in the area. Answers a and d would increase the weakness of the external rotators. Answer c would increase the contraction of the internal rotator.

25. **c**
Application and concept identification
Rationale: The question presents an example of a clinical reasoning process. Knowledge of the four-step process is necessary to answer the question. Brainstorming generates options.

26. **d**
Application and concept identification
Rationale: The question asks for intelligent application of methods with respect for existing compensation pattern. The client has resourceful compensation that was disturbed by the massage intervention.

27. **a**
Factual recall
Rationale: The terms need to be defined. Assessment must be quantified as much as possible. All of the possible answers would result in a measurement, but only answer a would identify connective tissue shortening.

28. **d**

    Application and concept identification
    Rationale: Evaluating a treatment plan is an
    analytical process that involves the use of the
    clinical reasoning model. One area that is
    considered is the feelings of the people involved,
    and this is the area being targeted by the
    question. Answers a and b are fact gathering,
    answer c is brainstorming. Only answer d
    indicates the feelings of the people involved,
    since compliance is all about feelings.

CHAPTER

23

Complementary Bodywork

Questions

1. *Bodywork methods that focus on meridians and points fall into which category?*

   a. Eastern and Oriental
   b. Reflex
   c. Energetic
   d. Structural

2. *A client has been receiving massage for a mild peripheral arterial circulation problem. Which of the following would be an appropriate self-help method to teach the client?*

   a. Lymphatic drainage
   b. Skin rolling
   c. Alternating applications of hot and cold
   d. Frictioning

3. *Cold applications of hydrotherapy to reduce swelling are called _____.*

   a. Analgesic
   b. Antipyretic
   c. Antispasmodic
   d. Antiedemic

4. *The secondary effect of a local cold application is _____.*

   a. Sedative
   b. Increased localized circulation
   c. Diaphoretic
   d. Decreased systemic circulation

5. *What is the water temperature for a neutral bath?*

   a. 65 to 92 degrees
   b. 98 to 104 degrees
   c. 92 to 98 degrees
   d. 56 to 65 degrees

6. *A folded towel soaked in water of the desired temperature and placed on a large area of skin is called a _____.*

   a. Tonic friction
   b. Vaporizer
   c. Sponge
   d. Pack

7. *RICE applications for first aid are appropriate for _____.*

   a. Primary care of abrasion
   b. Grade 2 and 3 sprains and strains
   c. Neural injury
   d. Shock

8. *A client has mild edema in her lower legs from a long plane flight the previous day. Which of the following is an appropriate treatment plan?*

   a. Short light gliding strokes focused on the legs. Compression to the soles of the feet. Active and passive joint movement for the ankle, knee, and hip. Placing the legs above the heart.

   b. Compression to the legs focused on the medial side from proximal to distal. Muscle energy and lengthening combined with stretching in the area of the most accumulation of fluid.

   c. Deep gliding strokes from proximal to distal on the legs. Placing the legs above the heart. Limiting movement to encourage drainage.

   d. Superficial and deep compression along the vessels in the lateral leg. Active resistive joint movement combined with shaking.

9. *A client is getting ready to play a tournament tennis game in 60 minutes. She wants to increase circulation and prepare her muscles for the game. Which of the following treatment plans in the best option?*

   a. Long gliding strokes from distal to proximal focused toward the heart combined with rocking. Duration of the massage—45 minutes.

   b. Broad-based compression to the soft tissue of the limbs generally focused from proximal to distal combined with shaking and tapotement. Duration of the massage—20 minutes.

   c. Full-body massage with muscle energy methods and lengthening. Duration of the massage—45 minutes.

   d. Compression, superficial myofascial release, and trigger point work focused on the limbs combined with passive joint movement and shaking. Duration of the massage—15 minutes.

10. *Because of a skin condition, general massage is contraindicated for a client, but he is allowed to have his feet and hands worked on. He complains of neck stiffness. If using foot reflexology theory, where would the massage practitioner focus massage on the foot to affect the neck?*

    a. Heel
    b. Tips of the toes
    c. Base of the large toe
    d. Sole of the foot

11. *Reflexology can be beneficial because _____.*

    a. The complex structure of the foot is highly innervated and sensitive to changes in pressure and position, making it highly responsive to massage manipulation

    b. The flexor withdrawal mechanism of the foot is inhibited with pressure to the foot, and this inhibits neural activity in the dorsal horn of the spinal cord

    c. The specific mapped areas of reflex activity in the foot to organs have a direct relationship to visceral/cutaneous responses

    d. Stimulation of the zone therapy points on the bottom of the foot activates meridian energy movement in the chakra system

12. *A client injured his right shoulder 3 years ago. Assessment indicates decreased mobility of the skin surrounding the shoulder coupled with a painful but normal range of motion. Which is the best treatment option for this client?*

    a. Deep transverse friction
    b. Superficial myofascial release
    c. Compression
    d. Lymphatic drainage

13. *Myofascial methods are most specifically focused on change in the _____.*

    a. Motor point
    b. Lymph nodes
    c. Gait control mechanism
    d. Ground substance

14. *Deep transverse friction applied correctly will* _____.

    a. Inhibit circulation
    b. Create controlled inflammation
    c. Provide broad-based application
    d. Replace broadening contractions

15. *Which of the following is correct in application of trigger point therapy?*

    a. 15-minute application in combination with lengthening and stretching
    b. 45-minute application with hydrotherapy cold applications
    c. Limiting application to active trigger points only
    d. Using pressure methods first and limiting lengthening

16. *An active trigger point that is left untreated for 6 months often will* _____.

    a. Become an ashi point
    b. Become hot to the touch
    c. Have fibrotic changes
    d. Only elicit referred pain

17. *Trigger points are commonly located in* _____.

    a. Ligaments
    b. Tendons
    c. The joint capsule
    d. Muscles

18. *When treating trigger points,* _____.

    a. Direct pressure methods and squeeze methods should be used first
    b. Positional release with lengthening is the first application method
    c. Connective tissue stretching needs to accompany muscle energy application
    d. Lengthening of the tissue housing the trigger point is only effective with a local tissue stretch

19. *In Shiatsu the points are called* _____.

    a. Hara
    b. Meridians
    c. Jitsu
    d. Tsubo

20. *In Shiatsu a Ki energy flow that is under energy is called* _____.

    a. Tao
    b. Kyo
    c. Jitsu
    d. AhShi

21. *In yin/yang theory, if yang is over energy, which is correct?*

    a. Meridians are in balance
    b. Stimulate yin and sedate yang
    c. Sedate yin and stimulate yang
    d. Apply acupressure to Jitsu points

22. *Which of the following meridians is yin?*

    a. Gallbladder
    b. Stomach
    c. Lung
    d. Large intestine

23. *Which of the following meridians is located on the lateral side of the body beginning at the ear and ending at the toes?*

    a. Pericardium
    b. Bladder
    c. Liver
    d. Gallbladder

24. *Which of the following meridians is most medial?*

    a. Central
    b. Spleen
    c. Liver
    d. Large intestine

Answers are on pages 168–170.

25. A client is experiencing pain on palpation of many points along the kidney meridian. Which element of the five elements contains the kidney meridian?

    a. Fire
    b. Water
    c. Wood
    d. Earth

26. Which is a correct way to sedate a hyperactive acupuncture point?

    a. Tap the point
    b. Vibrate the point
    c. Place sustained pressure on the point
    d. Stimulate the meridian containing the point

27. In the earth element, if the stomach is yang, then what is yin?

    a. Spleen
    b. Bladder
    c. Liver
    d. Triple heater

28. Going clockwise on the five-element wheel, which element is adjacent to the fire element?

    a. Earth
    b. Metal
    c. Water
    d. Wood

29. In the five-element theory, what is the relationship of water to fire?

    a. Yin
    b. Yang
    c. Inhibiting
    d. Facilitating

30. A client has a cough and nasal mucus, diarrhea, and intestinal cramping. The large intestine meridian is tender to the touch. Which other meridian that is part of the metal element is directly involved?

    a. Pericardium
    b. Lung
    c. Bladder
    d. Heart

31. A system of health and medicine developed in India is called _____.

    a. Prana
    b. Elements
    c. Polarity
    d. Ayurveda

32. Which of the following is considered an Ayurvedic dosha?

    a. Pitta
    b. Marma
    c. Governing
    d. Ch'I

33. In Ayurvedic theory, bones, flesh, skin, and nerves belong to which element?

    a. Ether
    b. Air
    c. Earth
    d. Water

34. A dosha is physiologically a/n _____.

    a. Nerve pathway
    b. Chemical pattern
    c. Electrical pattern
    d. Dietary pattern

35. A client complains of increased hunger and thirst, feels hot, and has been in a bad temper lately. Which of the Ayurvedic elements is out of balance?

    a. Earth
    b. Fire
    c. Water
    d. Ether

36. In Ayurveda, the chakras are considered _____.

    a. Seven centers of prana located in the aura
    b. Seven centers of ki located on the central meridian
    c. Seven centers of prana located along the spinal column
    d. Six locations of kyo corresponding to centers of consciousness

37. *Massage in Ayurvedic theory concentrates on* _____.

    a. Manipulation of the doshas
    b. Tapping, rubbing, and squeezing points called kapha
    c. Movement of fluid along the vata centers
    d. Tapping, rubbing, and squeezing points on the body called marmas

38. *A system that combines the theory of Oriental medicine and Ayurveda is* _____.

    a. Polarity
    b. Rolfing
    c. Shiatsu
    d. Reflexology

39. *The main therapeutic focus of polarity therapy is to* _____.

    a. Balance the tridosha system
    b. Restore balance in the yin/yang system
    c. Remove structural imbalance
    d. Locate blocked energy and release it

40. *In polarity theory, the left side of the body is considered* _____.

    a. Ether
    b. Negative
    c. Neutral
    d. Positive

41. *In polarity theory, how many major body currents exist?*

    a. Two
    b. Three
    c. Five
    d. Seven

42. *In polarity theory, the color green is associated with which body current?*

    a. Ether
    b. Air
    c. Fire
    d. Water

43. *If an area of blocked energy is located, a simple polarity method is to* _____.

    a. Place the left hand on the painful area and the right hand opposite the painful area
    b. Rub the area with specialized oil preparations
    c. Press into the area with the fire finger and hold
    d. Stimulate the corresponding marma

44. *In polarity therapy, the joints are considered* _____.

    a. Chakra areas
    b. Serpentine brain wave currents
    c. Neutral
    d. Negative

45. *In polarity therapy, the heel of the foot is in a reflex relationship with the* _____.

    a. Shoulders and chest
    b. Pelvis
    c. Head and brain
    d. Abdomen

Answers are on pages 168–170.

Answers and Discussion

1. **a**
   Factual recall
   Rationale: The terms need to be defined to identify the correct answer.

2. **c**
   Application and concept identification
   Rationale: The key to this question is self-help. The one approach that most lends itself to this is hydrotherapy.

3. **d**
   Factual recall
   Rationale: The terms need to be defined to identify the correct answer.

4. **b**
   Factual recall
   Rationale: The question describes an effect of cold after the primary effect.

5. **c**
   Factual recall
   Rationale: The terms need to be defined to identify the correct answer.

6. **d**
   Factual recall
   Rationale: The terms need to be defined to identify the correct answer.

7. **b**
   Application and concept identification
   Rationale: The question asks first for a definition of RICE to be able to identify when it is most appropriate. Then the possible answers need to be defined to correlate the best answer with the recommended application of rest, ice, compression, and elevation.

8. **a**
   Clinical reasoning/synthesis
   Rationale: The facts presented in the question present a logical explanation for mild edema. The question asks for safe and beneficial treatment application. Knowledge about anatomy, physiology, and physiologic effect of massage methods is necessary to choose the correct answer. The correct answer describes the recommended combination of methods to support normal lymphatic function. The incorrect answers present either misinformation or less effective application of methods.

9. **b**
   Clinical reasoning/synthesis
   Rationale: Accumulated knowledge is necessary to answer the question. The main focus is increasing arterial blood flow without interfering with performance. Any massage over 30 minutes would be fatiguing, which eliminates answers a and c. Any work that would substantially change muscle tone or create pain is contraindicated prior to athletic performance, so the only logical answer is answer b.

10. **c**
    Factual recall
    Rationale: The question asks for the area on the foot that would affect the condition based on reflexology theory.

11. **a**
    Factual recall
    Rationale: The correct answer provides a scientific explanation for the benefits of foot massage.

12. **b**
    Application and concept identification
    Rationale: All of the methods presented as possible answers need to be defined and then analyzed for best application based on the information in the question. Deep transverse friction is too aggressive. Compression and lymphatic drain are likely to be less effective than the correct answer, which is superficial myofascial release.

13. **d**
    Factual recall
    Rationale: All the terms need to be defined to identify ground substance as the correct answer.

14. **b**
    Factual recall
    Rationale: The correct answer describes the physiologic effect of deep transverse friction, controlled inflammation.

15. **a**
    Factual recall
    Rationale: Muscles containing trigger points need to be lengthened to restore normal resting length. No more than 15 minutes of this type of intervention is recommended.

16. **c**
Application and concept identification
Rationale: The changes that occur when a condition such as trigger points becomes chronic instead of acute involve fibrotic changes.

17. **d**
Factual recall
Rationale: Trigger points are found in muscles.

18. **b**
Application and concept identification
Rationale: Recommendation of treatment of trigger points is to use least invasive measures first. The wrong answers are either too aggressive (answers a and c) or misinformation (answer d).

19. **d**
Factual recall
Rationale: This question is an example of how terminology describing Eastern and Oriental methods can be presented in text questions. All the terms need to be defined.

20. **b**
Factual recall
Rationale: This question is an example of how terminology describing Eastern and Oriental methods can be presented in text questions. All the terms need to be defined.

21. **b**
Application and concept identification
Rationale: The relationship of yin to yang needs to be understood along with all the terminology to identify the correct answer. In yin/yang theory over energy is sedated and under energy is stimulated.

22. **c**
Factual recall
Rationale: All terms need to be defined and the meridians categorized as yin or yang to answer the question.

23. **d**
Factual recall
Rationale: The location of all the meridians would need to be identified to answer the question.

24. **a**
Factual recall
Rationale: The location of all the meridians would need to be identified to answer the question.

25. **b**
Factual recall
Rationale: The relationship of the meridians to the five elements is necessary to answer the question.

26. **c**
Application and concept identification
Rationale: The question is asking for the application that would calm down an acupuncture point. The three wrong answers would result in increased energy in the point.

27. **a**
Factual recall
Rationale: The relationships of the meridians to the five elements are necessary to answer the question.

28. **a**
Factual recall
Rationale: The relationships of the five elements to each other are necessary to answer the question.

29. **c**
Application and concept identification
Rationale: The metaphor of the five elements for the qualities represented by fire and water would indicate that water inhibits fire.

30. **b**
Factual recall
Rationale: Lung and large intestine make up the metal element.

31. **d**
Factual recall
Rationale: Define the terms to identify the correct answer.

32. **a**
Factual recall
Rationale: Define the terms to identify the correct answer.

33. **c**
Factual recall
Rationale: The physiology represented by the Ayurvedic elements needs to be defined to answer the question.

34. **b**
Factual recall
Rationale: The relationships of the dosha to physiology need to be defined to answer the question.

35. **b**
    Application and concept identification
    Rationale: The question is representative of how many questions can be developed to test knowledge about complementary bodywork. Each of the Ayurvedic elements needs to be defined to identify the symptoms that would indicate dysfunction.

36. **c**
    Factual recall
    Rationale: The question is testing terminology. The incorrect answers are not part of the language used in Ayurveda or present incorrect information.

37. **d**
    Factual recall
    Rationale: All the terminology needs to be defined to identify the answer that makes sense. A dosha is a chemical pattern, not a physical part of the body to be massaged. The marmas are points on the body.

38. **a**
    Factual recall
    Rationale: This is a definition question.

39. **d**
    Factual recall
    Rationale: The wrong answers describe modalities other than polarity.

40. **b**
    Factual recall
    Rationale: The right side is positive energy flow and the left side is negative energy flow.

41. **c**
    Factual recall
    Rationale: Five currents exist—ether, air, fire, water, earth.

42. **b**
    Factual recall
    Rationale: Each body current has a color sense, food, and other qualities. These need to be understood to answer the question.

43. **a**
    Application and concept identification
    Rationale: Polarity theory indicates that placing a negative energy flow over the pain and a positive energy flow opposite the pain will move and balance the energy.

44. **c**
    Factual recall
    Rationale: The flexibility of the joints indicates that they are neutral.

45. **b**
    Factual recall
    Rationale: Study a diagram to identify foot reflexes in the polarity system.

CHAPTER

24

Serving Special Populations

Questions

1. *In which area would additional study be required when working with any population with special needs?*

   a. Massage methods
   b. Special situations
   c. Psychology
   d. Relaxation methods

2. *An adult male client has many surgical scars on his chest and abdomen. History indicates that the client had surgical intervention as a child to repair congenital malformations. The client enjoys massage on the limbs and back in the prone position but appears distant and unsettled when turned to the supine position. What is the most logical explanation for this response?*

   a. An abusive family history
   b. Reenactment
   c. Dissociation
   d. Integration

3. *A college football player is seeking massage as part of a healing program for an injured knee that required surgical intervention. The athletic trainer is supervising the massage. The massage consists of general full-body massage that addresses any developing compensation caused by the gait change while the knee is healing. Specific applications of kneading and myofascial release are being used to maintain pliability in the soft tissue of the upper and lower leg. What type of massage is being performed?*

   a. Postevent massage
   b. Recovery massage
   c. Remedial massage
   d. Rehabilitation massage

4. *In which of the following circumstances would breast massage be most appropriate?*

   a. General massage
   b. Adjunct to breast cancer treatment
   c. Scar tissue management
   d. Examination for lumps

5. *In which of the following circumstances would massage without supervision by a health care professional best benefit children?*

   a. Growing pains
   b. Anxiety disorder
   c. Touch sensitivity
   d. Attention deficient disorder

6. *A massage professional has been working with a client who has chronic pain syndrome. The massage helps when combined with physical therapy, judicious use of pain medications, and support group attendance. Improvement in the condition begins after six or seven massage sessions. After ten to twelve sessions the client misses three or four sessions, then returns for massage and indicates that she is right back where she started. She states that she doesn't feel like the situation will ever improve. What is the most logical explanation for this behavior?*

   a. State-dependent memory
   b. Decrease in hardiness
   c. Secondary gain
   d. Acute pain

7. *What would be the most challenging counter-transference situation a massage professional faces when working with clients with chronic illness?*

   a. Understanding combined effects of massage and medications
   b. Managing frustration with a client whose condition does not improve
   c. Maintaining boundaries with a client who sees massage as the answer to all physical problems
   d. Managing acute episodes of chronic illness

8. *A massage professional has been working with an 86-year-old female client. The client still lives independently with some outside support. Family lives in a nearby state. The client is unable to drive. In which way does this client most likely benefit from a weekly massage?*

   a. Physical and emotional stimulation
   b. Increased circulation
   c. Friendship
   d. Spiritual support

9. *A parent massaging their infant encourages _____.*

   a. Hardiness
   b. Dissociation
   c. Developmental disabilities
   d. Bonding

10. *A massage therapist has just started a job at a family practice medical center. The center deals with many clients who exhibit stress-related symptoms. Which of the following professional skills will the massage therapist need to perfect?*

    a. Muscle energy methods
    b. Restorative massage
    c. Charting and record keeping
    d. Lymphatic drainage

11. *A client just began working with a massage professional who specializes in massage for those with physical disability. Which of the following would be a likely accommodation the client would notice?*

    a. The building is barrier free
    b. Special massage methods are used
    c. All client have guardians
    d. All clients set quantifiable and qualifiable goals

12. *A massage practitioner has been asked by a group of mental health professionals to begin working at a residential facility. She would need to be most concerned over which of the following?*

    a. Types of mental health issues
    b. Obtaining informed consent
    c. Learning specific massage protocols for each condition
    d. Frequency and duration of the massage

13. *A massage therapist has developed a referral network with a group of physicians and physiologists dealing with anxiety and panic disorders. Which of the following will he need to be effective in managing with massage?*

    a. Exercise protocols
    b. Nutrition
    c. Support group interactions
    d. Hyperventilation syndrome

14. *A massage client is in the first trimester of her third pregnancy. Which of the following is contraindicated?*

    a. Prone position
    b. Massage of the feet
    c. Deep abdominal massage
    d. Lymphatic drainage

15. *A long-term client has just notified you that he has a terminal illness. Which of the following can massage best offer?*

    a. Therapeutic change
    b. Palliative care
    c. Remedial massage
    d. Rehabilitation massage

Answers and Discussion

1. **b**
   Factual recall
   Rationale: Massage methods do not change but the people being served do.

2. **c**
   Application and concept identification
   Rationale: The question describes dissociation and provides a logical explanation for why the client might respond in such a way.

3. **d**
   Application and concept identification
   Rationale: The client is an athlete, so the approach is sports massage. Sports massage has categories of treatment that need to be defined to answer the question.

4. **c**
   Application and concept identification
   Rationale: Ethical concerns exist for breast massage for the female client. Scar tissue massage is the most relevant form of massage to the breast area.

5. **a**
   Clinical reasoning/synthesis
   Rationale: Each of the conditions listed needs to be defined and then analyzed in relationship to massage for children without the supervision of a medical professional. Answers b, c, and d are more complex conditions than growing pains.

6. **c**
   Clinical reasoning/synthesis
   Rationale: The question describes a pattern often seen in those with chronic pain. As soon as improvement is seen, clients seem to sabotage themselves. In such a situation secondary gain may be present.

7. **b**
   Application and concept identification
   Rationale: The terms need to be defined. Dealing with those with chronic pain can cause frustration for the massage professional.

8. **a**
   Factual recall
   Rationale: For many, massage is the professional structure for human contact.

9. **d**
   Factual recall
   Rationale: Pleasurable and secure touch supports bonding.

10. **c**
    Factual recall
    Rationale: Working with special populations in a health care setting requires special attention to record keeping.

11. **a**
    Factual recall
    Rationale: The most common accommodation for those with physical disability is barrier-free access to the facility.

12. **b**
    Application and concept identification
    Rationale: With mental health issues, the ability of the client to make an informed decision is a priority.

13. **d**
    Factual recall
    Rationale: A common factor that can be managed with massage in this population is breathing in excess of demand, which triggers a sympathetic nervous system dominance pattern contributing to the anxiety symptoms.

14. **c**
    Factual recall
    Rationale: The three trimesters of pregnancy need to be defined to identify the correct answer in relation to massage application.

15. **b**
    Factual recall
    Rationale: The terms in the question and possible answers need to be defined to identify the correct answer.

25

Wellness Education

Questions

1. *During the massage a client often speaks of problems with his children respecting house rules. This is a _____.*

   a. Body issue
   b. Mind issue
   c. Spiritual issue
   d. Core issue

2. *A massage practitioner notices that he becomes a bit aloof if he gets behind and is late for scheduled massage sessions. This is a/n _____.*

   a. Denial measure
   b. Defensive measure
   c. Exhaustion phase response
   d. Lack of purpose

3. *Wellness programs usually include methods to improve communication. Which of the following best explains why communication is more difficult to improve than diet?*

   a. Diet and nutrition are more concrete and objective than subjective communication
   b. Diet is much more dependent on others while communication is independent of others
   c. Stress focuses change toward healthy food choices
   d. Communication skills are highly genetically influenced but diet is not

4. *Wellness usually involves simplification of lifestyle to reduce demands. A stressful outcome of this process is often _____.*

   a. Hyperventilation syndrome
   b. Financial stability
   c. Dealing with loss and letting go
   d. Increased social support

5. *When breathing in the normal relaxed pattern, _____.*

   a. The inhale is longer than the exhale
   b. Deep inspiration is accentuated
   c. Accessory muscles only work on exhalation
   d. The exhale is longer than the inhale

6. *When one is considering the wellness components of balanced body, mind, and spirit, in which of the following intervention areas is massage most effective?*

   a. Promoting exercise
   b. Restoration of an appropriate eating and sleep cycle
   c. Normalization of breathing mechanisms
   d. Promoting belief system changes

Answers are on page 177.   **175**

7. *A client feels fatigued all the time. She explains that she doesn't seem to sleep all night. Which of the following may improve her situation?*

   a. An afternoon cup of coffee
   b. Taking a long nap in the afternoon
   c. Going to bed and watching television
   d. Spending at least 30 minutes outdoors

8. *When one feels confident with commitment, control, and challenge in life, one is _____.*

   a. Coping well
   b. Using behavior modification
   c. Functioning from an external locus of control
   d. Reliant on defense mechanisms

Answers and Discussion

1. **b**
   Factual recall
   Rationale: The question provides an example of mind issues.

2. **b**
   Factual recall
   Rationale: The question provides an example of defensive measures.

3. **a**
   Application and concept identification
   Rationale: All three of the wrong answers present incorrect information. The strategy in developing the incorrect answers is to pair conflicting statements together. The correct answer states a logical connection.

4. **c**
   Factual recall
   Rationale: The reduction of demand means letting go of something to lighten the stress load.

5. **d**
   Factual recall
   Rationale: The entire breathing cycle needs to be understood to answer the question. Only the correct answer presents correct breathing when relaxed.

6. **c**
   Application and concept identification
   Rationale: Massage cannot do everything. Wellness is multidimensional. While massage can support various lifestyle changes, it can directly influence breathing function.

7. **d**
   Factual recall
   Rationale: Various activities can either support or interfere with sleep patterns. The three wrong answers can interfere with sleep.

8. **a**
   Factual recall
   Rationale: The question defines effective coping.

CHAPTER

26

Business Considerations for a Career in Therapeutic Massage

Questions

1. *A massage professional is considering a position at a local day spa. The owner of the business offered either an employee position at a salary or a subcontractor position based on commission. Which would be an advantage of the employee position?*

   a. Variable income
   b. Stable income
   c. Subject to employer's regulations
   d. Independent ability to set work hours

2. *A massage professional has been working 12-hour days, 6 days a week, for 2 years. She is seeing 40 clients per week. Lately she finds herself tired and out of sorts. She does not attempt to rebook clients who cancel. What is the most logical explanation for her behavior?*

   a. Motivation
   b. Coping mechanisms
   c. Burnout
   d. Infection

3. *Expenses used to begin new business operations are called _____.*

   a. Business plan
   b. Reimbursement
   c. Investments
   d. Start-up costs

4. *A massage therapist is involved with developing a promotional campaign to increase his massage business since taking on a part-time massage employee. What is this called?*

   a. Marketing
   b. Business plan
   c. Resume
   d. Management

5. *A massage practitioner has just redesigned his brochure and has included the types of massage provided, what the massage is like, information about the practitioners' qualifications, and client responsibilities. What did he forget?*

   a. Tax structures
   b. Type of premise liability insurance
   c. Fees
   d. Client-practitioner agreement

6. *A client notices that the massage office is clean, neat, and efficient and that licenses and certifications are posted on the wall. The client is impressed with the massage practitioner's abilities in _____.*

   a. Applications of massage
   b. Communication skills
   c. Marketing
   d. Management

7. *A massage professional wants to check to see if the location for an office being considered for rental is in an appropriate business distinct. Where does one find this information?*

   a. Local zoning office
   b. Facility rental agreement
   c. State licensing bureau
   d. County clerk's office

8. *Gross income minus expenses equals _____.*

   a. Deductions
   b. Deposits
   c. Net income
   d. A draw

9. *The type of insurance needed to protect in case a client falls while in the business location is _____.*

   a. Malpractice
   b. Premise liability
   c. Independent contractor liability
   d. Disability

10. *A massage practitioner has obtained required licenses for her business location. The type of business set up was a sole proprietorship with a DBA. She has her business checking account and tax plan developed with an attorney. She also contacted a local insurance agent for appropriate insurance. She is a member of a professional organization that supplies professional liability insurance. She has a marketing plan and client practitioner agreements. What did she forget?*

    a. Retirement investment plan
    b. Zoning approval
    c. Salary structure
    d. Business plan

Answers and Discussion

1. **b**
   Factual recall
   Rationale: Standard comparison of the two types of positions indicates that stable income is considered an advantage.

2. **c**
   Application and concept identification
   Rationale: When considering all the information provided in the question against the implications of the possible answer, burnout seems the most likely situation.

3. **d**
   Factual recall
   Rationale: As with all questions of this type, the terminology needs to be defined to answer the question. The question is the definition of start-up costs.

4. **a**
   Factual recall
   Rationale: The question provides an example of marketing.

5. **c**
   Factual recall
   Rationale: The common elements included in a brochure need to be compared to the list provided in the question to identify the missing element.

6. **d**
   Factual recall
   Rationale: The question provides an example of management.

7. **a**
   Factual recall
   Rationale: The government department that deals with zoning would determine whether the business was in the proper district.

8. **c**
   Factual recall
   Rationale: The question is the definition of net income.

9. **b**
   Factual recall
   Rationale: The question defines premise liability insurance.

10. **a**
    Factual recall
    Rationale: All the components of a business plan have been identified in the question except for a retirement plan.

27

Integration Questions Covering Multiple Content

Questions

1. A massage professional is relocating the massage practice from a city to a rural area. The population is primarily farm workers and factory workers who commute to a nearby city. After interviewing some of the people from the town, the massage professional discovers that low back pain and fatigue are chief complaints and that the average income is $35,000 per year. Which combination of methods and marketing would be the best to quickly build the new business?

   a. General massage with energetic specialization provided in the client's home at a cost of $75 per session. Newspaper advertising used.

   b. General massage with myofascial and trigger point specialization in a one-person office. Massage rate set at $40 for a 1-hour massage, with an introductory offer of a free 30-minute massage when a package deal of five massage sessions is purchased for $150.

   c. A multiperson office providing space for three full-time massage practitioners and two part-time practitioners, with each practitioner having a particular specialty. Massage fees set at $55 per session. A radio campaign with $5 coupon offered.

   d. Subleasing a room in the local cosmetology business and providing general massage for relaxation. Fees set at $45 per session. Advertising done by word of mouth and free 15-minute chair massages on Saturdays.

2. A client had a severe viral infection 4 years ago and continues to have episodes of relapse. She has just recently been diagnosed with fibromyalgia. During assessment, the massage professional notices that the client inhales longer than she exhales and that most of the movement during breathing happens in the upper chest. Her physician has suggested massage as part of a total management program but is asking for a treatment plan. Which of the following is the most reasonable expectation in terms of benefit, cost, and compliance?

   a. Weekly massage for 3 months
   b. Monthly massage for 12 months
   c. Weekly massage indefinitely
   d. Massage three times a week for 6 months

3. A massage professional has experienced a substantial increase in client base in the last 3 months because of skills in soft-tissue mobilization with massage. He books 25 clients per week and has a waiting list of 15 clients wishing appointments. He has attempted to squeeze in an additional four or five clients by extending evening appointments. He charges $40 for a 1-hour massage. He nets $600 per week and would like to increase his income by $100 per week. During the last month he has been experiencing fatigue and mild shoulder pain, which disturbs him. One of the reasons he became a massage professional was to be able to work independently without personnel problems. Which of the following would be the best suggestion from a mentor?

   a. Raise prices by $5 per session and review application of body mechanics
   b. Increase client load by three clients and switch from general massage to energetic methods
   c. Raise prices by $10 and reduce client load to 20 clients
   d. Hire a massage practitioner and increase client load in the business by 15 clients

4. A client seeks massage to support parasympathetic dominance and reduce a tendency toward high blood pressure. The client responds best to applications of broad-based heavy compression or deep gliding strokes. Skin mobility and flexibility are good, as is range of motion. The client prefers to be nonparticipative during the massage. The client prefers weekly appointments in the evening. The massage professional has been working with this client for 3 months, and while the client is pleased with the work, the massage professional is exhausted after the session. What is the most likely cause?

   a. The client is emotionally draining and the therapist has issues with countertransference
   b. The massage professional finds the sessions complex and interactive, and the constant challenge is fatiguing
   c. The nonparticipation by the client is unrealistic in terms of client goals, requiring the massage professional to work too hard
   d. The client's needs are basic and nonchallenging and the therapist is using poor body mechanics to maintain the pressure and repetitive nature of the massage

5. A client is seeking reimbursement for massage fees from his insurance company. He was injured in a car accident and the massage is primarily palliative. He has requested a summary report from the massage therapist describing the massage care received over the past 6 months. Where will the massage professional obtain the data to write this report?

   a. Treatment plan
   b. Client history
   c. Informed consent
   d. SOAP charts

6. A client requested a relaxation massage. The client then complained that the massage felt uncomfortable and that the skin on her back was warm and itching. Postprocedure assessment indicated a histamine response midthorax, in the area between T-6 and T-12. Which of the following components of massage was incorrect in relation to the client's goals?

   a. Direction
   b. Drag
   c. Duration
   d. Rhythm

7. A massage professional is experiencing shoulder pain and has the sensation of tingling and numbness in the arms. The massage professional can identify various trigger points in the trapezius and scalenes when the area is palpated. The massage practice has doubled from 10 clients per week to 20 clients per week, and while she enjoys the increased income and is pleased to now have a full-time practice, she feels pressured to perform. Instead of relaxing at the end of the day, she feels anxious, restless, and fatigued. She also recognizes that she is breathing more shallowly and yawns often. Which of the following would be the best intervention?

   a. Reduce massage clients to 10 sessions per week and take a month sabbatical
   b. Reduce massage clients to 15 sessions per week and see her physician for antianxiety medication
   c. Have a peer check body mechanics to look for overuse of shoulder muscles and speak to her mentor about managing business pressures
   d. Raise rates so that 10 clients provide the same income as 20 clients

8. *A massage professional recently relocated the business to work in partnership with a mental health professional who refers patients for stress management. The massage practitioner is now required to write monthly reports on client progress and meet with the psychologist. The clients are progressing, and both the massage professional and the psychologist can observe the changes, but the reports provided are vague and confusing to the psychologist. Which of the following is the most likely cause?*

    a. Use of too many abbreviations in the narrative report

    b. Lack of pre- and postassessment in relation to quantitative and qualitative goals

    c. Ineffective informed consent procedures

    d. Subtle physiologic changes that cannot be measured

9. *A massage professional has been working with a college football player to increase endurance and reduce tendency toward muscle strains. The massage professional uses a combination of methods to influence muscle tone, connective tissue pliability, and fluid dynamics, particularly blood exchange in the capillary beds on the lower legs. The massage professional has recently taken a class on muscle energy methods and has been using them to lengthen the muscles of the athlete's legs. The athlete feels looser but his performance has decreased and the coach and athletic trainer are not pleased. They feel that something with the massage may be the cause. Which of the following would support the coach and athletic trainer's position?*

    a. The training effect on the leg muscles has been disrupted by the introduction of the muscle energy methods

    b. The massage has caused increased inflammation in the tissues

    c. The client is fatigued after participating in the muscle energy methods

    d. The massage professional has not performed the methods correctly

10. *A student of massage is preparing to take final examinations. She has been informed that the exam is comprehensive, timed, and multiple choice in design. She has been diligent in her studies and practicum and feels confident to begin working on clients once she graduates. She feels nervous about remembering all of the details she has studied, especially scientific terminology and clinical reasoning methods. She wants to be alert while taking the examination but not anxious. Which of the following would be good advice for this student?*

    a. Cram study just before the exam to make sure of all the terminology

    b. Drink coffee while studying to keep awake but not before the exam

    c. Breathe deeply with long inhale and short exhale patterns to decrease anxiety

    d. Get a massage the day before the exam, sleep well, and remember to exhale slowly while taking the exam.

Answers are on pages 188–189.

Answers and Discussion

1. **b**
   Clinical reasoning/synthesis
   Rationale: The question covers special populations issues, specific massage outcomes, methods of massage, complementary bodywork, and marketing. All the pieces have to come together to create a successful practice. The population is blue collar and would have to justify the cost versus benefit, especially since the average income is below $40,000 per year. The potential clients have typical low back pain and fatigue, which respond well to general massage and the more mechanical methods of myofascial and trigger point applications. The correct answer addresses these issues, while the business plan offered in the wrong answers would better serve a different population and target market.

2. **c**
   Clinical reasoning/synthesis
   Rationale: The question combines information about pathology, contagious diseases, assessment, breathing patterns, treatment plan development, and clinical reasoning skills. Each of the possible answers addresses frequency and duration of the massage, and the best choice for the condition listed is condition management, which would be based on weekly sessions indefinitely.

3. **a**
   Clinical reasoning/synthesis
   Rationale: Content covered includes business practices, motivation, massage skills and application, body mechanics, ethics and professional skills, and support by a mentor. All of the possible answers need to be evaluated against the information presented in the question. Answer a is the correct answer. Answer b is incorrect because it shifts methods from what is working to an unfamiliar form to the client base. Answer c is incorrect since the practitioner did not experience problems until he began to increase his workload, indicating that 25 appointments per week is manageable and a $10 raise may actually decrease clients. Answer d is incorrect because the massage professional states he does not want to work with anyone.

4. **d**
   Clinical reasoning/synthesis
   Rationale: Content covers anatomy and physiology, application and physiologic outcome of massage methods, assessment application and interpretation, business structure, body mechanics, professional dynamics and ethics, and burnout. The question asks about the condition of the massage professional in relationship to this client. Answer a is incorrect because the client is not emotionally draining. Answer b is incorrect because the session is based on repetitive application of basic skills. Answer c is incorrect because the goals are realistic. Answer d is correct because the massage professional is likely to be bored with the client and using poor body mechanics.

5. **d**
   Application and concept identification
   Rationale: Content covered is charting, insurance reimbursement, type of care, and content of a narrative summary. The SOAP notes best describe the ongoing care information necessary to write the narrative.

6. **b**
   Clinical reasoning/synthesis
   Rationale: Content covered is physiology of relaxation and methods used to achieve this outcome, histamine response symptoms and what would cause them, assessment, and analysis of effectiveness of methods used. The four answers present the qualities of massage. Since the client did not request connective tissue work, the drag was too intense for the outcome.

7. **c**
   Clinical reasoning/synthesis
   Rationale: Content covered is assessment, trigger points, muscle anatomy and physiology, business practices, body mechanics, and symptoms of hyperventilation. Self-care and a change in business structure are provided in the correct answer. The incorrect answers do not address the fact that the client likes what is being done. Only answer c provides information that pertains to the question.

8. **b**
   Clinical reasoning/synthesis
   Rationale: Content covered includes business environment, mental heath affiliation requirements, referral, stress response, record keeping, communication skills, justification process skills, development of quantitative and qualitative goals, and outcome measurement. The correct answer identifies the confusion related to unclear outcomes for the massage sessions.

9. **a**
   Clinical reasoning/synthesis
   Rationale: Content covered includes athletic population and massage approaches, outcomes, massage methods, physiologic effects, resourceful compensation patterns, and professional dynamics with supervising professionals. This question points out complex situations and the bigger picture in terms of massage application as presented in the correct answer.

10. **d**
    Clinical reasoning/synthesis
    Rationale: This question may be describing you. If you have been a committed student, used the textbooks as suggested, reviewed with this study guide, and have a heart's desire to do massage, it will all work out. There is no way you will remember everything. The goal is not to be perfect. It is to be a compassionate and skilled massage professional who continues to learn for a lifetime. Remember to take care of yourself, get a massage, breathe from your diaphragm instead of your chest, sleep, eat and relax prior to the exam, and put the whole process in perspective.

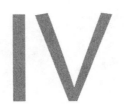

28

Labeling Exercises

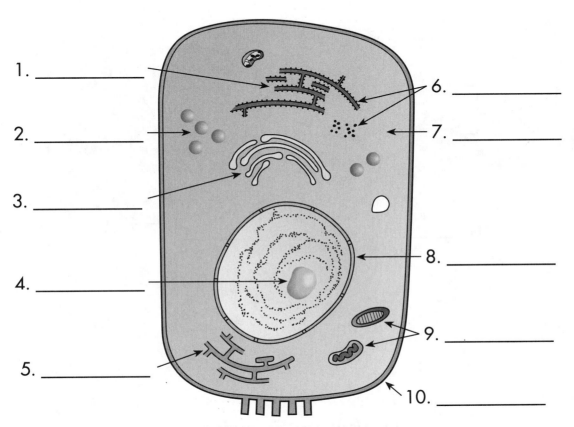

1. _____

2. _____

3. _____

4. _____

5. _____

6. _____

7. _____

8. _____

9. _____

10. _____

Labeling Exercise 1
Generalized Cell

Choices

Cell (plasma) membrane   Lysosome   Ribosomes
Cytoplasm   Mitochondria   Rough endoplasmic reticulum
Golgi apparatus   Nucleolus   Smooth endoplasmic reticlum
                          Nucleus

Modified from Williams RW: *Basic Healthcare Terminology*, St. Louis, 1995, Mosby
For use in Fritz: *Mosby's Massage Therapy Review*
Copyright © 2002, Mosby, *A Harcourt Health Sciences Company*

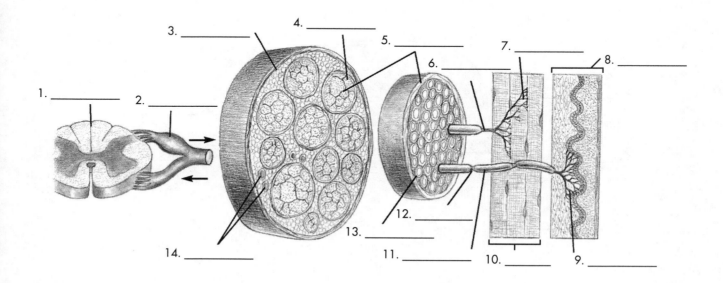

Labeling Exercise 2
Peripheral Nerve Trunk and Coverings

Choices

Axon	Muscle	Perineurium
Blood vessels	Myelin sheath	Skin
Endoneurium	Nerve bundle (fasciculus)	Spinal cord
Epineurium	Node of Ranvier	Spinal ganglion
Motor end plate	Pain receptors	

Answers are on pages 233–242.

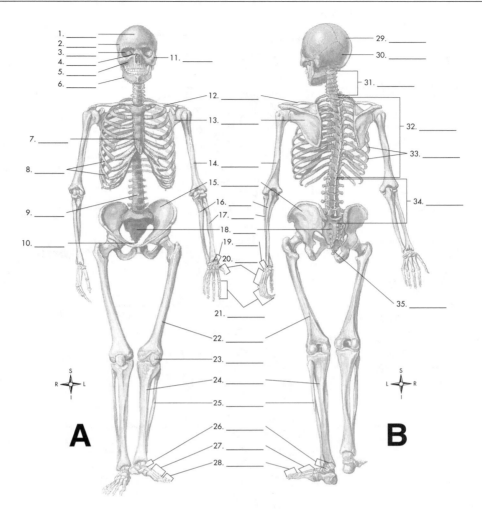

Labeling Exercise 3
Skeleton. A, Anterior view. B, Posterior view.

Choices

Carpals	Maxilla	Sacrum
Cervical vertebrae	Metacarpals	Scapula
Clavicle	Metatarsals	Skull
Coccyx (2 times)	Nasal bone	Sternum
Coxal (hip) bone	Occipital bone	Tarsals
Femur	Orbit	Thoracic vertebrae
Fibula	Parietal bone	Tibia
Frontal bone	Patella	Ulna
Humerus	Phalanges (2 times)	Vertebral column
Lumbar vertebrae	Radius	Zygomatic bone
Mandible	Ribs (2 times)	

Modified from Thibodeau GA, Patton KT: *Anatomy and Physiology*, ed 4, St. Louis, 1996, Mosby
For use in Fritz: *Mosby's Massage Therapy Review*
Copyright © 2002, Mosby, *A Harcourt Health Sciences Company*

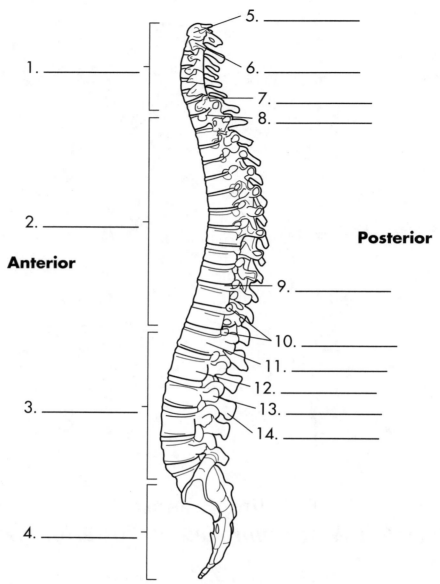

5. _____

6. _____

1. _____

7. _____

8. _____

2. _____

Anterior

Posterior

9. _____

10. _____

11. _____

12. _____

3. _____

13. _____

14. _____

4. _____

Labeling Exercise 4
Vertebral Column

Choices

Body	Intervertebral disk	Seventh cervical vertebra
Cervical curve	Intervertebral foramina	Spinous process
First cervical vertebra (atlas)	Lumbar curve	Thoracic curve
First lumbar vertebra	Sacral curve	Transverse process
First thoracic vertebra	Second cervical vertebra (axis)	

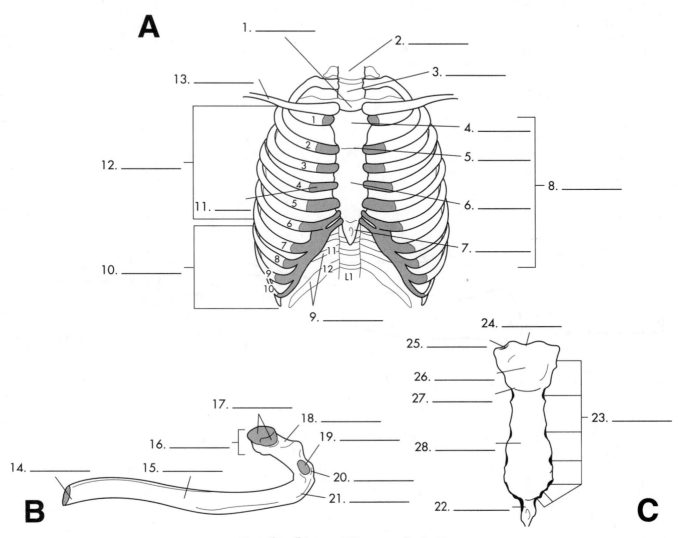

Labeling Exercise 5
A, Rib cage. B, Typical rib. C, Sternum

Choices

Angle
Articular facet for transverse
    process of vertebrae
Articular facets for body of
    vertebrae
Body (3 times)
Clavicle
Clavicular notch
Costal cartilage

Facets for attachment of costal
    cartilages 1 to 7
False ribs
First thoracic vertebra
Floating ribs
Head
Jugular notch (2 times)
Manubrium (2 times)
Neck

Seventh cervical vertebra
Sternal angle (2 times)
Sternal end
Sternum
True ribs
Tubercle
Xiphoid process (2 times)

For use in Fritz: *Mosby's Massage Therapy Review*
Copyright © 2002, Mosby, *A Harcourt Health Sciences Company*

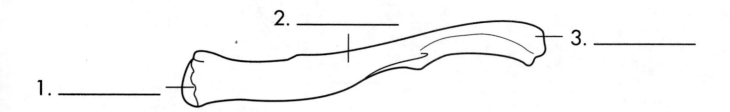

2. _____

3. _____

1. _____

Labeling Exercise 6
Clavicle

Choices

Acromial end
Body
Sternal end

For use in Fritz: *Mosby's Massage Therapy Review*
Copyright © 2002, Mosby, *A Harcourt Health Sciences Company*

Answers are on pages 233–242.

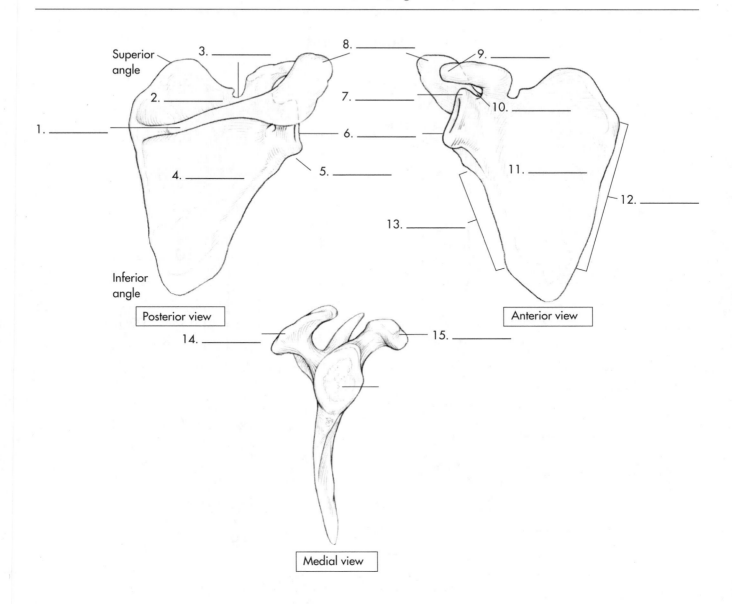

Superior angle

3.

2.

1.

4.

Inferior angle

8.

7.

6.

5.

Posterior view

9.

10.

11.

12.

13.

Anterior view

14.

15.

Medial view

Labeling Exercise 7
Scapula: Three Views

Choices

Acromion	Infraspinous fossa	Supraglenoid tubercle
Coracoid fossa	Lateral border	Suprascapular notch
Coracoid process	Scapular spine (2 times)	Supraspinous fossa
Glenoid fossa (2 times)	Spinoglenoid notch	Vertebral border
Infraglenoid tubercle	Subscapular fossa	

Modified from Mathers LH et al: *Clinical anatomy principles,* St. Louis, 1996, Mosby
For use in Fritz: *Mosby's Massage Therapy Review*
Copyright © 2002, Mosby, *A Harcourt Health Sciences Company*

Answers are on pages 233–242.

Right Humerus

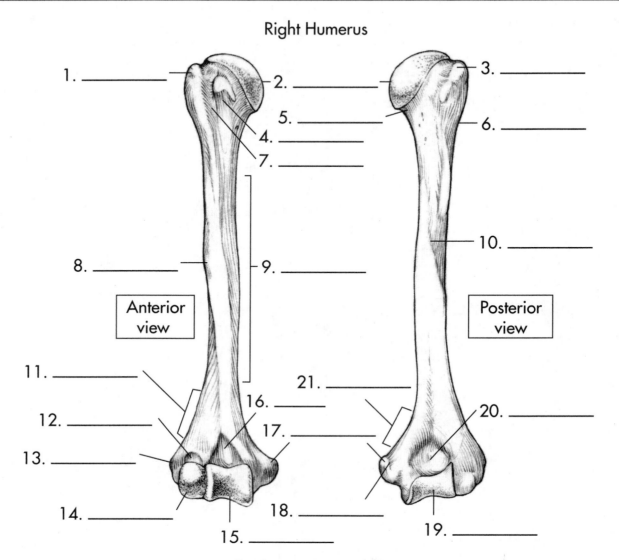

1. _____   2. _____
                  5. _____
                  4. _____
                  7. _____

3. _____
6. _____

8. _____   9. _____   10. _____

Anterior view

Posterior view

11. _____   16. _____
12. _____   17. _____
13. _____
14. _____   18. _____
15. _____

21. _____
20. _____
19. _____

Labeling Exercise 8
Humerus: Anterior and Posterior Views

Choices

Anatomic neck	Lateral epicondyle	Radial fossa
Capitulum	Lateral supracondylar ridge	Radial groove
Coronoid fossa	Lesser tubercle	Shaft of humerus
Deltoid tuberosity	Medial epicondylar groove	Surgical neck
Greater tubercle (2 times)	Medial epicondyle	Trochlea (2 times)
Head	Medial supracondylar ridge	
Intertubercular groove	Olecranon fossa	

Modified from Mathers LH et al: *Clinical anatomy principles,* St. Louis, 1996, Mosby
For use in Fritz: *Mosby's Massage Therapy Review*
Copyright © 2002, Mosby, *A Harcourt Health Sciences Company*

Answers are on pages 233–242

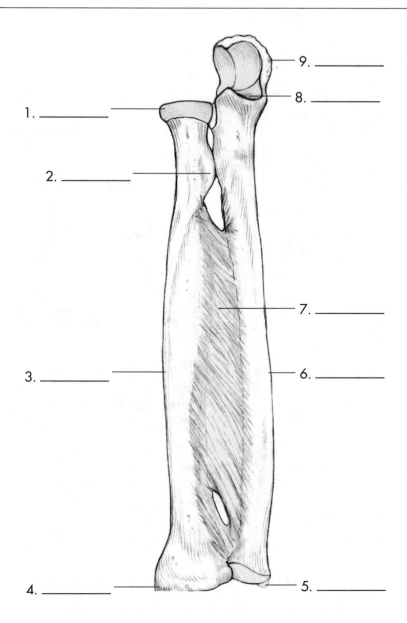

Labeling Exercise 9
Forearm Bones

Choices

Interosseous membrane	Radial styloid	Trochlear notch
Olecranon process of ulna	Radial tuberosity	Ulna
Radial head	Radius	Ulnar Styloid

Modified from Mathers LH et al: *Clinical anatomy principles*, St. Louis, 1996, Mosby
For use in Fritz: *Mosby's Massage Therapy Review*
Copyright © 2002, Mosby, *A Harcourt Health Sciences Company*

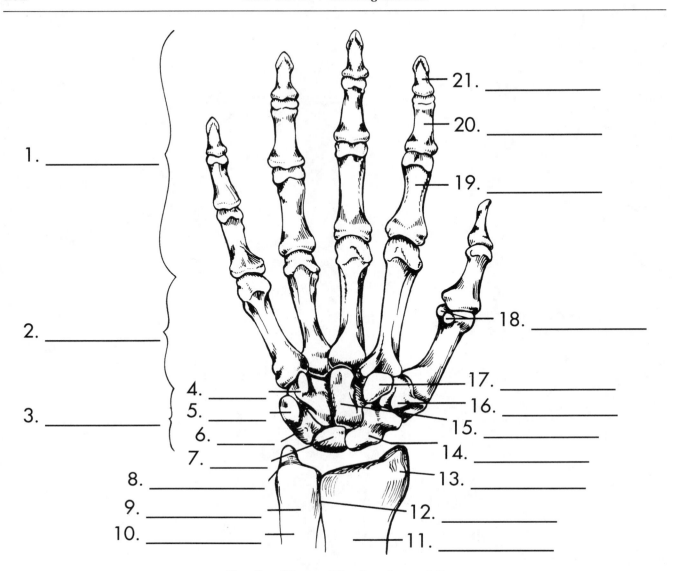

Labeling Exercise 10
Hand Skeleton: Volar View

Choices

Capitate	Phalanges	Trapezium
Carpus	Pisiform	Trapezoid
Distal	Proximal	Triquetrum
Hamate	Radius	Ulna
Lunate	Scaphoid	Ulnar head
Metacarpus	Sesamoids	Ulnar notch of radius
Middle	Styloid process (2 times)	

Modified from Malone TR, McPoil T, Nitz AJ: *Orthopedic and sports physical therapy,* ed 3, St. Louis, 1997, Mosby
For use in Fritz: *Mosby's Massage Therapy Review*
Copyright © 2002, Mosby, *A Harcourt Health Sciences Company*

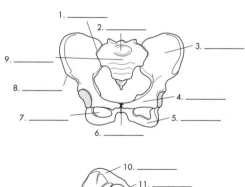

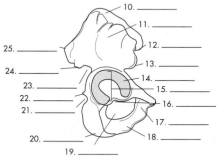

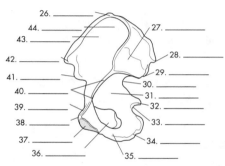

Labeling Exercise 11
Pelvis

Choices

Acetabular notch
Acetabulum
Anterior inferior iliac spine (2 times)
Anterior superior iliac spine (3 times)
Auricular surface
Body of ischium
Greater sciatic notch (2 times)
Iliac crest (2 times)
Iliac fossa

Iliopectineal line
Ilium (3 times)
Inferior pubic ramus (2 times)
Ischial ramus (2 times)
Ischial spine (2 times)
Ischial tuberosity
Ischium
Lesser sciatic notch (2 times)
Lunate surface
Obturator foramen (3 times)
Posterior inferior iliac spine (2 times)

Posterior superior iliac spine (2 times)
Pubic crest
Pubis
Sacral promontory
Sacroiliac joint
Sacrum
Superior pubic ramus
Symphysis pubis (2 times)

For use in Fritz: *Mosby's Massage Therapy Review*
Copyright © 2002, Mosby, *A Harcourt Health Sciences Company*

Answers are on pages 233–242.

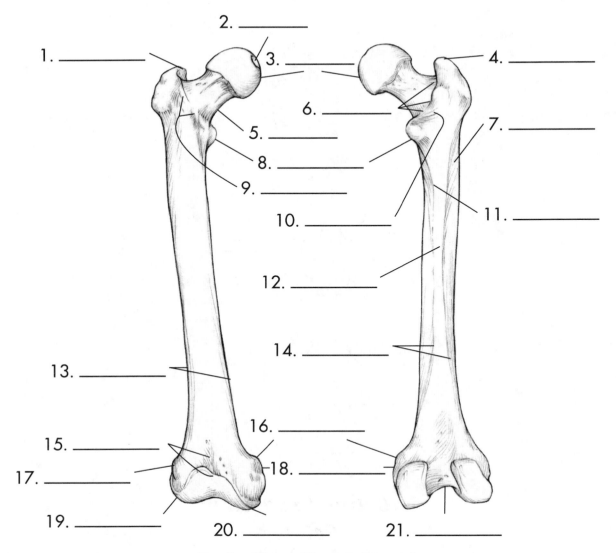

Labeling Exercise 12
Right Femur: Anterior and Posterior Views

Choices

Adductor tubercle	Intertrochanteric fossa	Medial and lateral supracondylar
Fovea capitis	Intertrochanteric line	lines
Gluteal tuberosity	Lateral and medial supracondylar	Medial condyle
Greater trochanter (2 times)	ridges	Medial epicondyle
Head of femur	Lateral condyle	Neck
Intercondylar fossa	Lateral epicondyle	Patellar groove
Intertrochanteric crest	Lesser trochanter	Pectineal line
	Linea aspera	

Modified from Mathers LH et al: *Clinical anatomy principles*, St. Louis, 1996, Mosby
For use in Fritz: *Mosby's Massage Therapy Review*
Copyright © 2002, Mosby, *A Harcourt Health Sciences Company*

Answers are on pages 233–242.

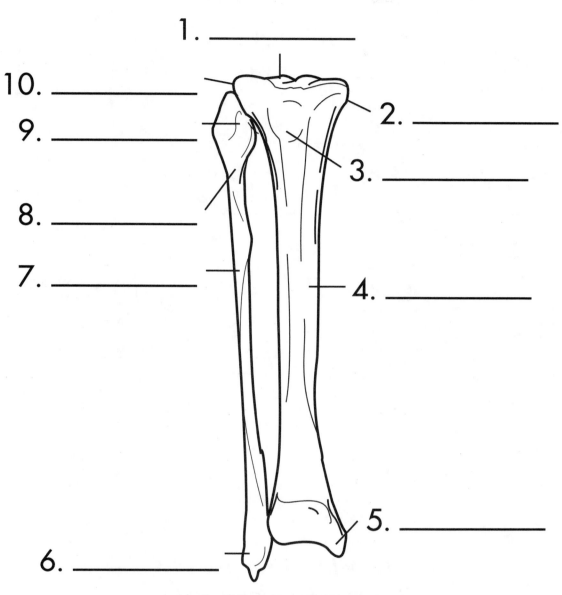

1. _____

10. _____

9. _____

8. _____

7. _____

6. _____

2. _____

3. _____

4. _____

5. _____

Labeling Exercise 13
Tibia and Fibula

Choices

Fibula	Lateral malleolus	Neck of fibula
Head	Medial condyle	Tibia
Intercondylar eminence	Medial malleolus	Tibial tuberosity
Lateral condyle		

For use in Fritz: *Mosby's Massage Therapy Review*
Copyright © 2002, Mosby, *A Harcourt Health Sciences Company*

Answers are on pages 233–242.

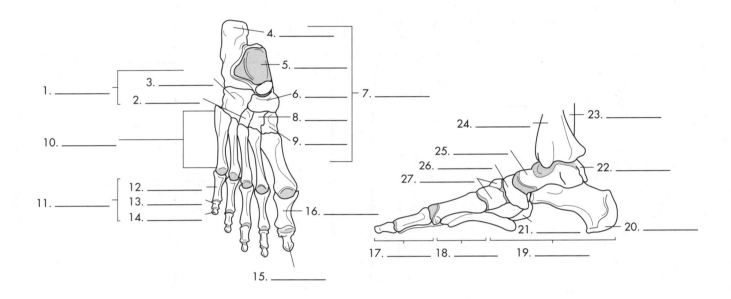

Labeling Exercise 14
Bones of Foot and Ankle

Choices

Calcaneus (2 times)
Cuboid (2 times)
Cuneiforms
Distal phalanx
Distal phalanx of great toe
Fibula

Intermediate cuneiform
Lateral cuneiform
Medial cuneiform
Metatarsals (2 times)
Middle phalanx
Navicular (2 times)

Phalanges (2 times)
Proximal phalanx
Proximal phalanx of great toe
Talus (3 times)
Tarsals (3 times)
Tibia

For use in Fritz: *Mosby's Massage Therapy Review*
Copyright © 2002, Mosby, *A Harcourt Health Sciences Company*

Answers are on pages 233–242.

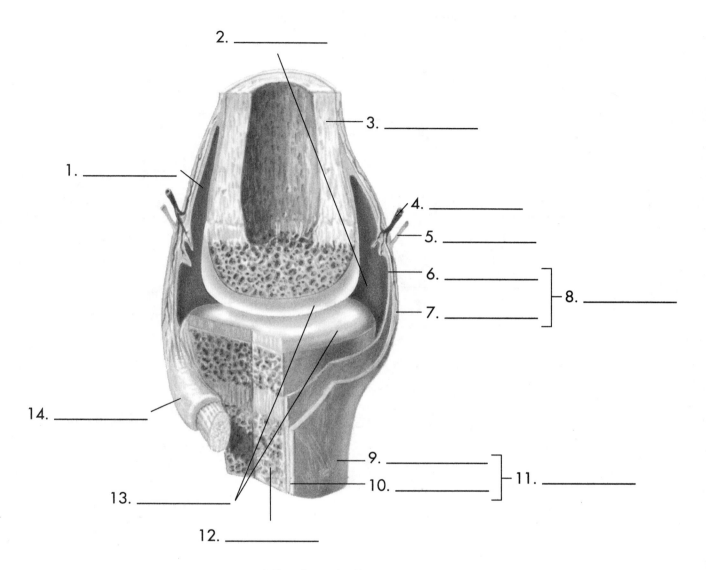

2. _____

3. _____

1. _____

4. _____

5. _____

6. _____

7. _____

8. _____

14. _____

9. _____

10. _____

11. _____

13. _____

12. _____

Labeling Exercise 15
Structures of a Synovial Joint (Knee)

Choices

Articular cartilage	Fibrous layer	Nerve
Blood vessel	Joint capsule	Periosteum
Bone (2 times)	Joint cavity (filled with synovial fluid)	Synovial membrane
Bursa		Tendon sheath
Fibrous capsule	Membranous layer	

Modified from Mourad LA: *Orthopedic disorders*, St. Louis, 1991, Mosby
For use in Fritz: *Mosby's Massage Therapy Review*
Copyright © 2002, Mosby, *A Harcourt Health Sciences Company*

Answers are on pages 233–242.

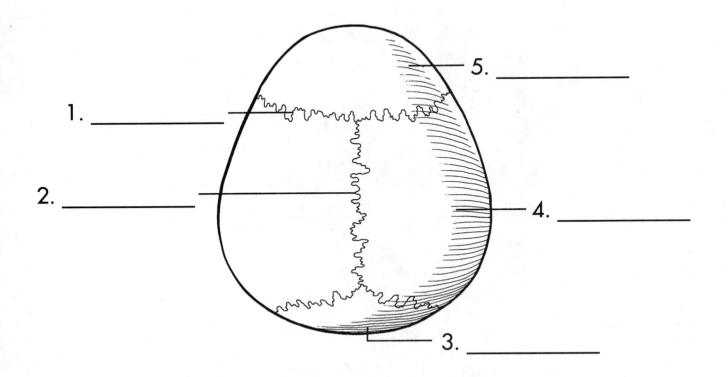

1. _____

2. _____

3. _____

4. _____

5. _____

Labeling Exercise 16
Skull: Top View

Choices

Coronal suture   Parietal bone
Frontal bone   Sagittal suture
Occipital bone

Modified from D'Ambrogio KJ, Roth GB: *Positional release therapy: assessment and treatment of musculoskeletal dysfunction*, St. Louis, 1997, Mosby
For use in Fritz: *Mosby's Massage Therapy Review*
Copyright © 2002, Mosby, *A Harcourt Health Sciences Company*

Answers are on pages 233–242.

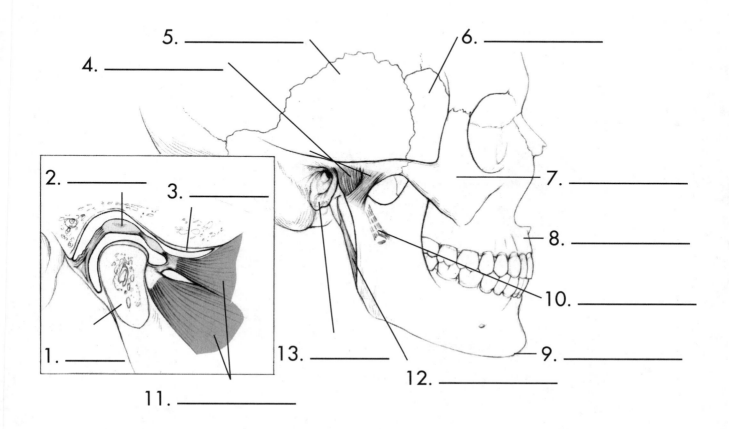

Labeling Exercise 17
Temporomandibular Joint and Inset of Articular Disk

Choices

Anterior tubercle, zygoma	Mandible	Temporal bone, squamous part
Articular disk	Maxilla	Two heads of lateral pterygoid muscle
Condylar process of mandible	Pterygomandibular septae	
External auditory meatus	Sphenoid, greater wing	Zygoma
Lateral temporomandibular ligament	Stylomandibular ligament	

Modified from Mathers LH et al: *Clinical anatomy principles,* St. Louis, 1996, Mosby
For use in Fritz: *Mosby's Massage Therapy Review*

Answers are on pages 233–242.

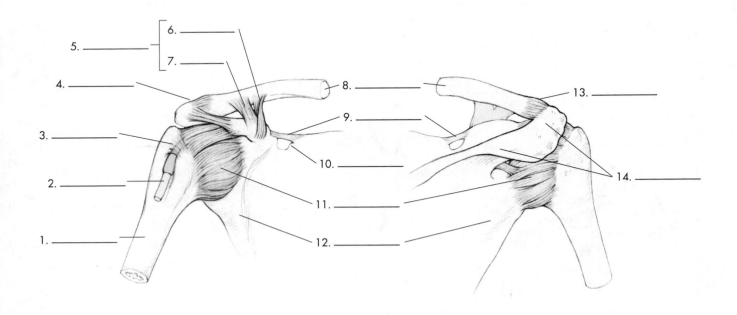

Labeling Exercise 18
Ligaments of Shoulder: Anterior and Posterior Views

Choices

Acromioclavicular ligament (2 times)	Glenohumeral ligament	Suprascapular notch
	Humerus	Transverse humeral ligament
Clavicle	Long head of biceps muscle	Transverse scapular ligament
Conoid ligament	Scapula	Trapezoid ligament
Coracoclavicular ligament	Scapular spine and acromion	

Modified from Mathers LH et al: *Clinical anatomy principles*, St. Louis, 1996, Mosby
For use in Fritz: *Mosby's Massage Therapy Review*
Copyright © 2002, Mosby, *A Harcourt Health Sciences Company*

Answers are on pages 233–242.

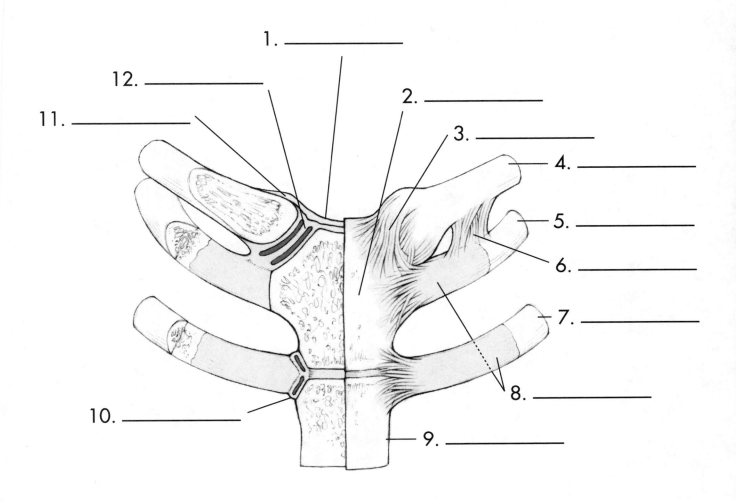

1. _____

12. _____

11. _____

2. _____

3. _____

4. _____

5. _____

6. _____

7. _____

8. _____

9. _____

10. _____

Labeling Exercise 19
Joints of Sternum

Choices

Articular disk   Costoclavicular ligament   Second rib
Body of sternum   First rib   Sternoclavicular joint
Clavicle   Interclavicular ligament   Sternoclavicular ligament
Costal cartilages   Manubrium of sternum   Synovial chondrosternal joint

Answers are on pages 233–242.

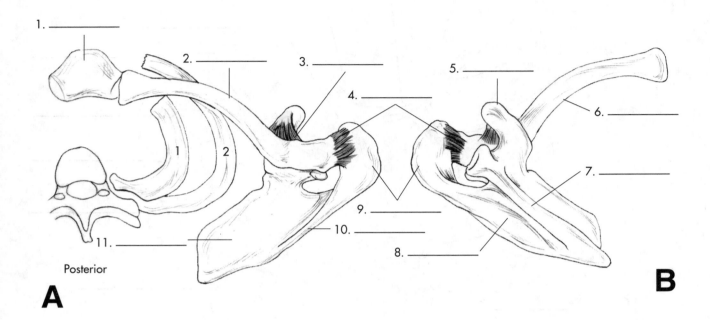

Posterior

A

B

Labeling Exercise 20
Acromioclavicular Joint of Shoulder Girdle.
A, Superior view. B, Inferior view.

Choices

Acromioclavicular ligament	Coracoid process	Scapular spine
Acromion	Inferior border of scapula	Sternum
Clavicle (2 times)	Infraspinous fossa	Subscapular fossa
Coracoclavicular ligament		

Modified from Mathers LH et al: *Clinical anatomy principles*, St. Louis, 1996, Mosby
For use in Fritz: *Mosby's Massage Therapy Review*

Answers are on pages 233–242.

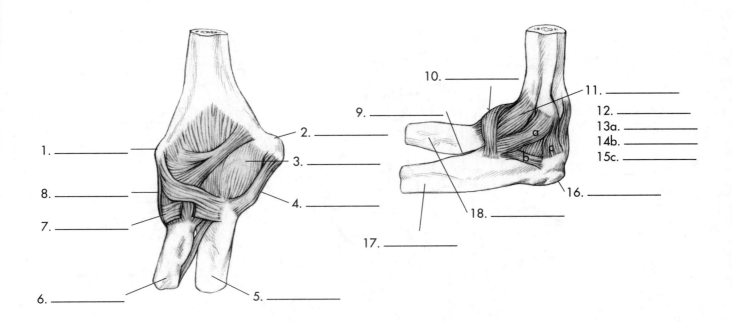

Labeling Exercise 21
Ligaments of Elbow Joint: Anteroposterior and Lateral Views

Choices

Annular ligament
Annular ligament of radius
Anterior band
Anterior elbow capsule
Elbow joint capsule
Lateral epicondyle

Medial epicondyle
Medial (ulnar) collateral ligament
Oblique band
Olecranon of ulna
Posterior band
Radial collateral ligament

Radial tuberosity
Radius (2 times)
Ulna (2 times)
Ulnar collateral ligament

Modified from Mathers LH et al: *Clinical anatomy principles,* St. Louis, 1996, Mosby
For use in Fritz: *Mosby's Massage Therapy Review*
Copyright © 2002, Mosby, *A Harcourt Health Sciences Company*

Answers are on pages 233–242.

BONES   JOINTS

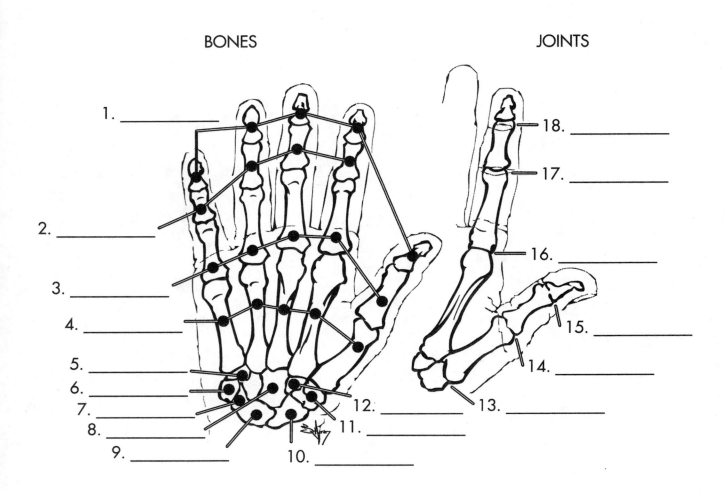

Labeling Exercise 22
Joints of Hand and Wrist

Choices

Capitate	Lunate	Proximal interphalangeal (PIP)
Carpometacarpal	Metacarpals	Proximal phalanges
Distal interphalangeal (DIP)	Metacarpophalangeal	Scaphoid
Distal phalanges	Metacarpophalangeal (MCP)	Trapezoid
Hamate	Middle phalanges	Trapezium
Interphalangeal	Pisiform	Triquetrum

Modified from Brister SJ: *Mosby's comprehensive physical therapist assistant board review*, St. Louis, 1996, Mosby
For use in Fritz: *Mosby's Massage Therapy Review*
Copyright © 2002, Mosby, *A Harcourt Health Sciences Company*

Answers are on pages 233–242.

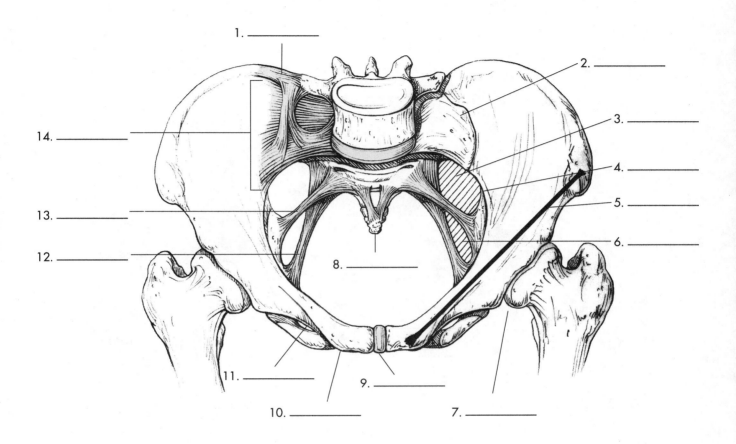

Labeling Exercise 23
Pelvic Ligaments: Superoanterior View

Choices

Acetabulum

Arcuate line

Coccyx

Greater sciatic foramen

Iliolumbar ligament

Inguinal ligament

Lesser sciatic foramen

Pectineal line

Pubic symphysis

Pubic tubercle

Sacroiliac joint

Sacroiliac ligament

Sacrospinous ligament

Sacrotuberous

Modified from Mathers LH et al: *Clinical anatomy principles,* St. Louis, 1996, Mosby
For use in Fritz: *Mosby's Massage Therapy Review*
Copyright © 2002, Mosby, *A Harcourt Health Sciences Company*

Answers are on pages 233–242.

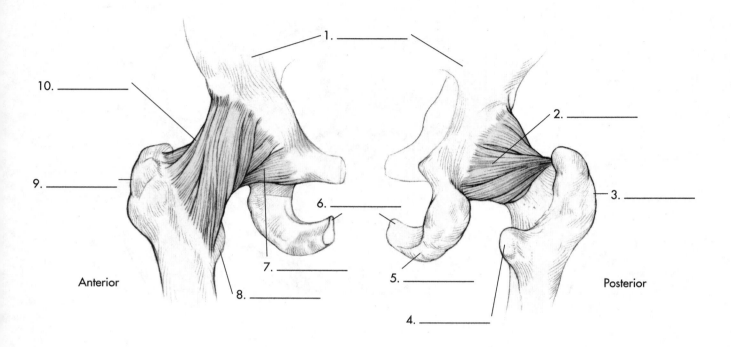

Labeling Exercise 24
Ligaments of Hip Joint

Choices

Greater trochanter (2 times)	Ischial tuberosity
Iliofemoral ligament	Ischiofemoral ligament
Ilium	Lesser trochanter (2 times)
Inferior pubic ramus	Pubofemoral ligament

Modified from Mathers LH et al: *Clinical anatomy principles,* St. Louis, 1996, Mosby
For use in Fritz: *Mosby's Massage Therapy Review*
Copyright © 2002, Mosby, *A Harcourt Health Sciences Company*

Answers are on pages 233–242.

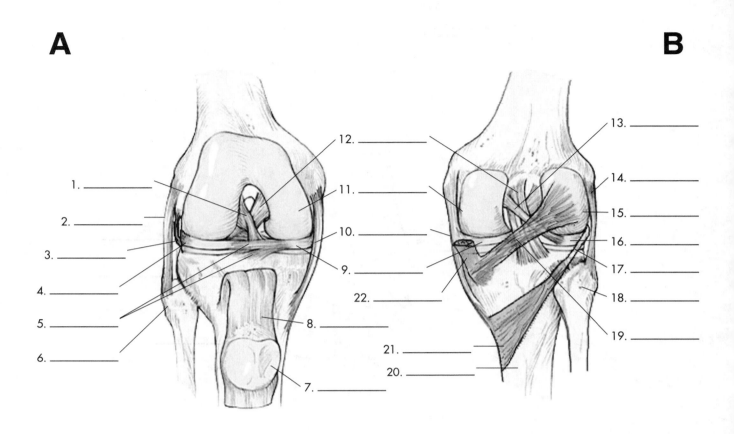

Labeling Exercise 25
Knee Joint Opened. A, Anterior view. B, Posterior view.

Choices

Anterior cruciate ligament
Fibular collateral ligament
Fibular head (2 times)
Fibular (lateral) collateral
    ligament
Lateral condyle
Lateral meniscus (2 times)
Medial condyle

Medial meniscus
Oblique popliteal ligament
Patella
Patellar ligament
Popliteus muscle
Popliteus tendon
Posterior cruciate ligament

Posterior meniscus femoral
    ligament
Semimembranous tendon
Tendon of popliteus muscle
Tibia
Tibial (medial) collateral ligament
Transverse ligament

Answers are on pages 233–242.

Medial view

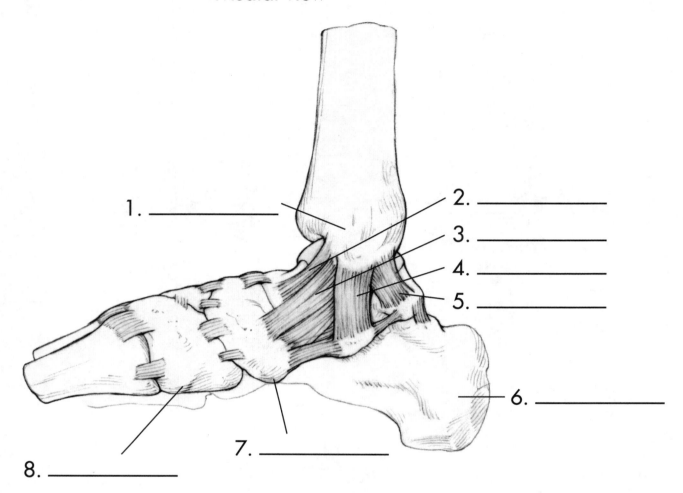

1. _____

2. _____

3. _____

4. _____

5. _____

6. _____

7. _____

8. _____

Labeling Exercise 26
Deltoid Ligament

Choices

Anterior tibiotalar	Navicular
Calcaneus	Posterior tibiotalar
Medial cuneiform	Tibiocalcaneal
Medial malleolus	Tibionavicular

Answers are on pages 233–242.

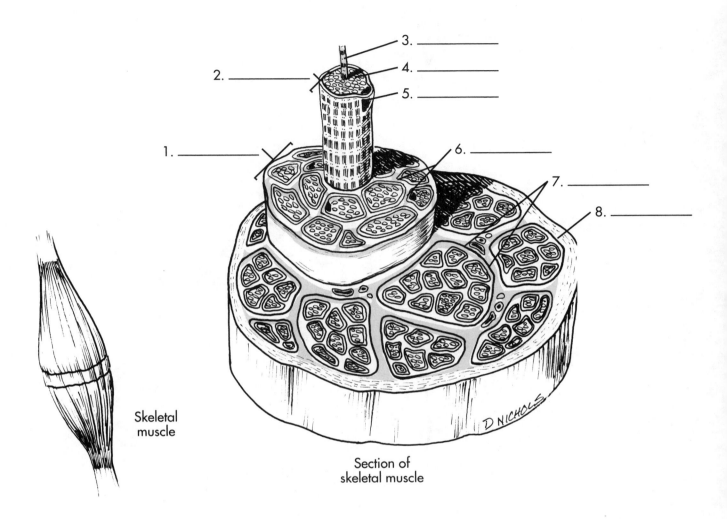

Skeletal
muscle

Section of
skeletal muscle

D NICHOLS

Labeling Exercise 27
Section of Skeletal Muscle with Contractile and Noncontractile Connective Tissue

Choices

Endomysium	Myofibril
Epimysium	Nucleus
Fascicle	Perimysium
Muscle fiber	Sarcolemma

Modified from Shankman GA: *Fundamental orthopedic management for the physical therapist assistant,* St. Louis, 1997, Mosby
For use in Fritz: *Mosby's Massage Therapy Review*
Copyright © 2002, Mosby, *A Harcourt Health Sciences Company*

Answers are on pages 233–242.

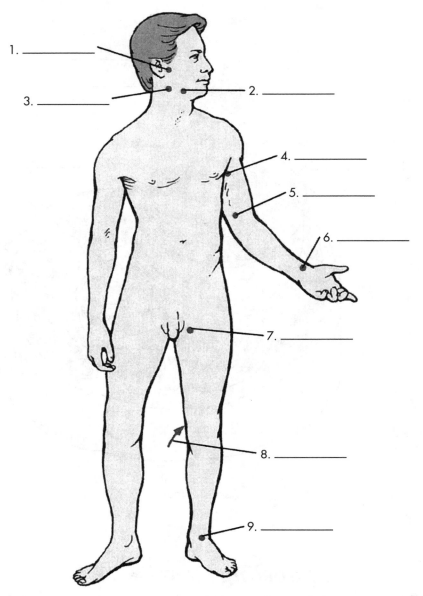

1. _____

3. _____

2. _____

4. _____

5. _____

6. _____

7. _____

8. _____

9. _____

Labeling Exercise 28
Pulse Points

Choices

Axillary artery   Dorsalis pedis artery   Popliteal artery
Brachial artery   Facial artery   Radial artery
Common carotid artery   Femoral artery   Superficial temporal artery

Modified from Thibodeau GA, Patton KT: *The human body in health and disease*, St. Louis, 1992, Mosby
For use in Fritz: *Mosby's Massage Therapy Review*
Copyright © 2002, Mosby, *A Harcourt Health Sciences Company*

Answers are on pages 233–242.

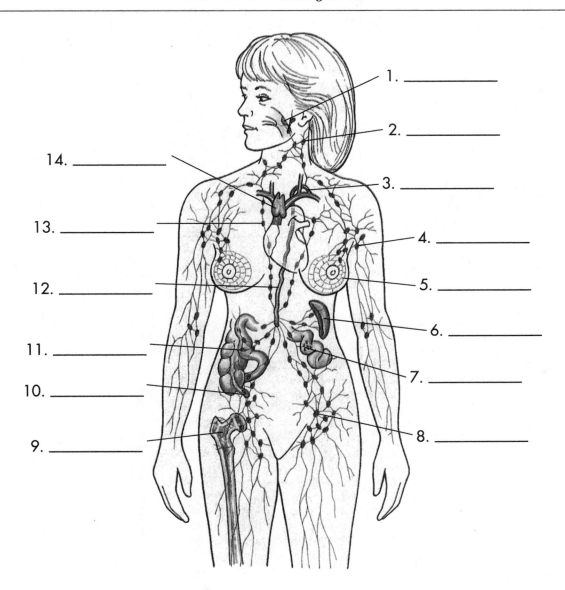

Labeling Exercise 29
Major Organs and Vessels of Lymphatic System

Choices

Appendix

Axillary lymph node

Bone marrow

Cervical lymph node

Entrance of thoracic duct into
   subclavian vein

Inguinal lymph nodes

Intestinal lymph nodes

Mammary plexus

Peyer's patches in intestinal wall

Right lymphatic duct

Spleen

Thoracic duct

Thymus gland

Tonsils

Modified from Seeley RR, Stephens TD, Tate P: *Anatomy and physiology,* St. Louis, 1995, Mosby
For use in Fritz: *Mosby's Massage Therapy Review*
Copyright © 2002, Mosby, *A Harcourt Health Sciences Company*

Answers are on pages 233–242.

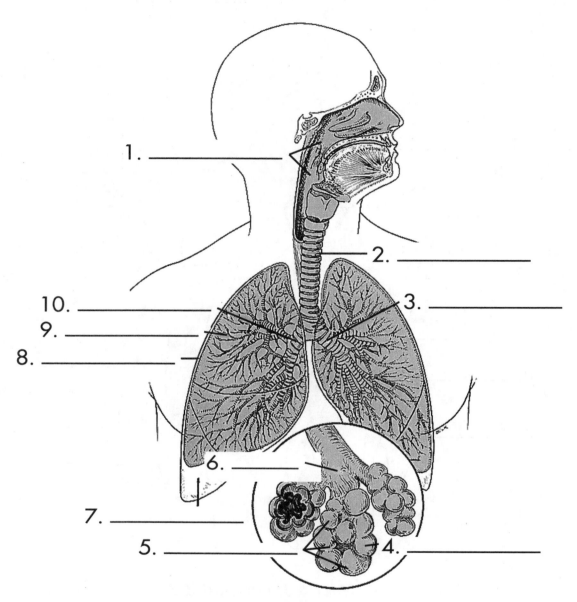

Labeling Exercise 30
Pharynx, Trachea, and Lungs, with Alveolar Sacs in Inset

Choices

Alveolar duct	Left main bronchus	Pleural space
Alveolar sac	Pharynx	Right main bronchus
Alveolus	Pleura	Trachea
Bronchiole		

Answers are on pages 233–242.

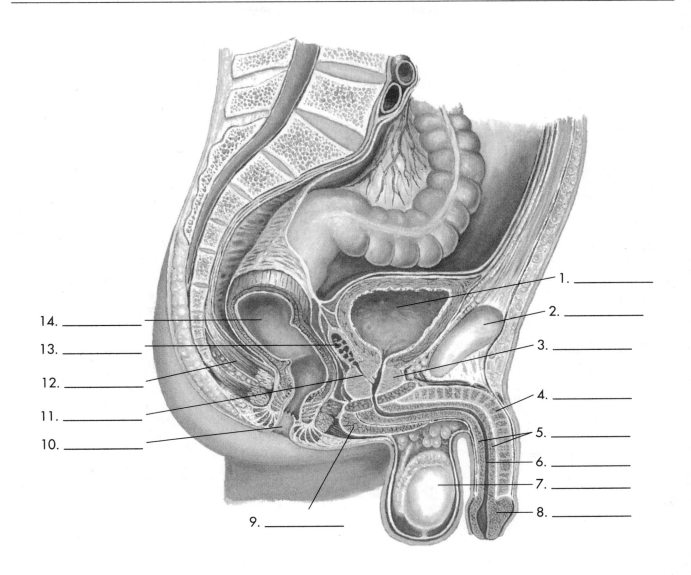

1. _____

2. _____

3. _____

4. _____

5. _____

6. _____

7. _____

8. _____

9. _____

14. _____

13. _____

12. _____

11. _____

10. _____

Labeling Exercise 31
Male Pelvic Organs

Choices

Anus	Glans	Symphysis pubis
Bulbocavernosus muscle	Levator ani muscle	Testis
Corpus cavernosum	Prostate gland	Urethra
Corpus spongiosum	Rectum	Urinary bladder
Ejaculatory duct	Seminal vesicle	

Answers are on pages 233–242.

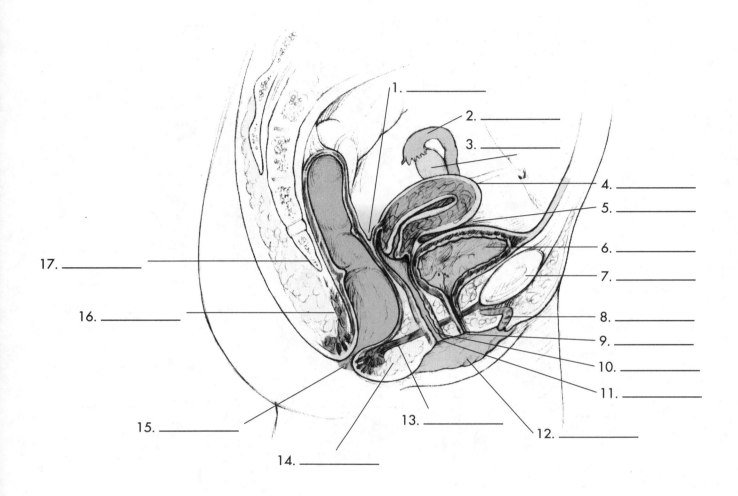

Labeling Exercise 32
Female Pelvic Floor: Midsagittal View

Choices

Anal orifice	Ovary	Urogenital diaphragm
Anococcygeal raphe	Oviduct	Uterus
Bladder	Perineal body	Vagina
Clitoris	Pubic symphysis	Vaginal introitus
Coccyx	Rectouterine fossa	Vesicouterine fossa
Labium minus	Urethral orifice	

Modified from Mathers LH et al: *Clinical anatomy principles,* St. Louis, 1996, Mosby
For use in Fritz: *Mosby's Massage Therapy Review*
Copyright © 2002, Mosby, *A Harcourt Health Sciences Company*

Answers are on pages 233–242.

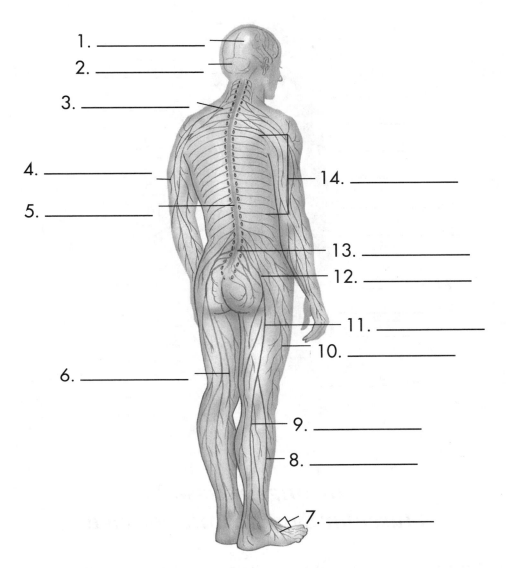

1. _____
2. _____
3. _____
4. _____
5. _____
6. _____
7. _____
8. _____
9. _____
10. _____
11. _____
12. _____
13. _____
14. _____

Labeling Exercise 33
Nervous System: Simplified View

Choices

Brachial plexus
Cauda equina
Cerebellum
Cerebrum
Digital nerves

Femoral cutaneous nerve
Femoral nerve
Intercostal nerves
Ischial nerve
Musculocutaneous nerve

Perineal nerve
Saphenous nerve
Spinal cord
Tibial nerve

Modified from LaFleur-Brooks M: *Exploring medical language: a student-directed approach,* ed 4, St. Louis, 1998, Mosby
For use in Fritz: *Mosby's Massage Therapy Review*
Copyright © 2002, Mosby, *A Harcourt Health Sciences Company*

Answers are on pages 233–242.

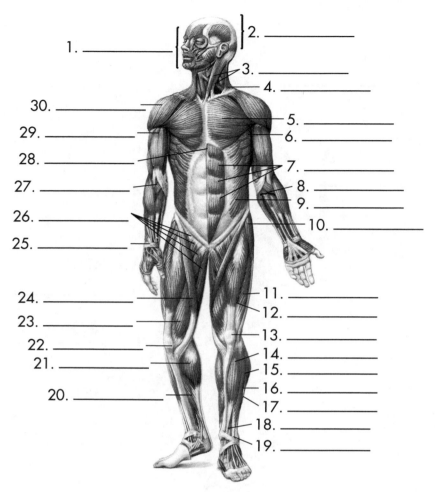

1. _____
2. _____
3. _____
4. _____
5. _____
6. _____
7. _____
8. _____
9. _____
10. _____
11. _____
12. _____
13. _____
14. _____
15. _____
16. _____
17. _____
18. _____
19. _____
20. _____
21. _____
22. _____
23. _____
24. _____
25. _____
26. _____
27. _____
28. _____
29. _____
30. _____

Labeling Exercise 34
Muscular System: Anterior View

Choices

Adductors of thigh	Gastrocnemius	Sartorius
Biceps brachii	Linea alba	Serratus anterior
Cranial muscles	Obliquus externus	Soleus
Deltoideus	Patella	Sternocleidomastoideus
Extensor digitorum longus	Patellar tendon	Superior extensor retinaculum
Extensor hallucis longus tendon	Pectoralis major	Tensor fasciae latae
Extensors of wrist and fingers	Peroneus brevis	Tibialis anterior
Facial muscles	Peroneus longus	Trapezius
Flexor retinaculum	Rectus abdominis	Vastus lateralis
Flexors of wrist and fingers	Rectus femoris	Vastus medialis

Modified from LaFleur-Brooks M: *Exploring medical language: a student-directed approach,* ed 4, St. Louis, 1998, Mosby
For use in Fritz: *Mosby's Massage Therapy Review*
Copyright © 2002, Mosby, *A Harcourt Health Sciences Company*

Answers are on pages 233–242.

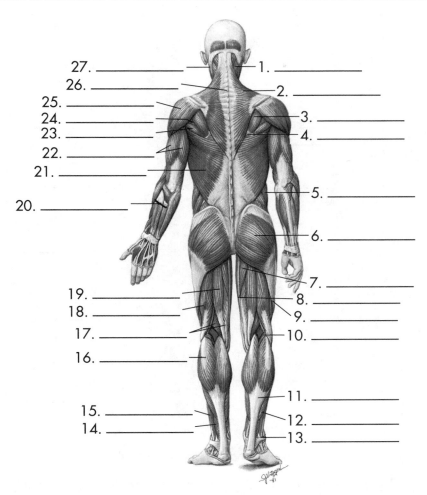

27. _____   _____ 1. _____
26. _____   2. _____
25. _____
24. _____   3. _____
23. _____   4. _____
22. _____
21. _____

20. _____   5. _____

                             6. _____

                             7. _____
19. _____   8. _____
18. _____   9. _____
17. _____   10. _____
16. _____

15. _____   11. _____
14. _____   12. _____
                            13. _____

Labeling Exercise 35
Muscular System: Posterior View

Choices

Adductor magnus	Infraspinatus	Seventh cervical vertebra
Biceps femoris	Latissimus dorsi	Soleus
Deltoideus	Obliquus externus	Splenius capitis
Extensors of the wrist and fingers	Peroneus brevis	Sternocleidomastoideus
Gastrocnemius	Peroneus longus	Superior peroneal retinaculum
Gastrocnemius tendon (Achilles tendon)	Plantaris	Teres major
Gluteus maximus	Portion of rhomboideus	Teres minor
Gracilis	Semimembranosus	Trapezius
Iliotibial tract	Semitendinosus	Triceps

Modified from LaFleur-Brooks M: *Exploring medical language: a student-directed approach*, ed 4, St. Louis, 1998, Mosby
For use in Fritz: *Mosby's Massage Therapy Review*
Copyright © 2002, Mosby, *A Harcourt Health Sciences Company*

Answers are on pages 233–242.

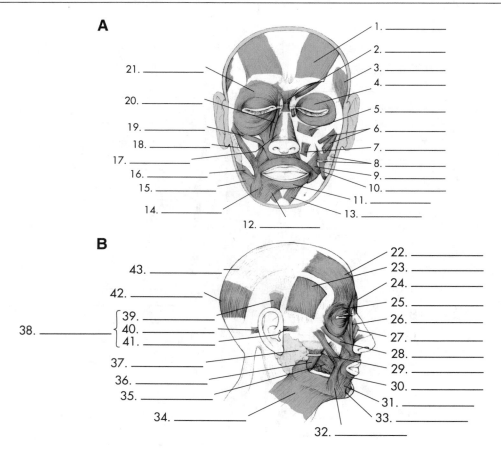

A

1. _____
2. _____
3. _____
4. _____
5. _____
6. _____
7. _____
8. _____
9. _____
10. _____
11. _____
13. _____
12. _____
14. _____
15. _____
16. _____
17. _____
18. _____
19. _____
20. _____
21. _____

B

22. _____
23. _____
24. _____
25. _____
26. _____
27. _____
28. _____
29. _____
30. _____
31. _____
33. _____
32. _____
34. _____
35. _____
36. _____
37. _____
38. _____
39. _____
40. _____
41. _____
42. _____
43. _____

Labeling Exercise 36
Facial Muscles. A, Anterior view. B, Lateral view.

Choices

Anterior
Auricular muscles
Buccinator muscle (2 times)
Depressor anguli oris
Depressor anguli oris muscle
Depressor labii inferioris (2 times)
Frontalis muscle (2 times)
Galea aponeurotica
Levator anguli oris
Levator labii superioris
Levator labii superioris alaeque
  nasi muscle (2 times)
Masseter muscle (2 times)

Mentalis
Mentalis muscle
Nasalis
Nasalis muscle
Occipitalis muscle
Orbicularis oculi muscle
Orbicularis oculi muscle
  (palpebral part)
Orbicularis oculi (orbital part)
Orbicularis oris muscle (2 times)
Parotid gland and duct (2 times)
Platysma
Platysma muscle

Posterior
Procerus muscle (2 times)
Risorius
Superior
Temporalis muscle (2 times)
Zygomaticus major muscle (2
  times)
Zygomaticus minor muscle (2
  times)
Zygomaticus major and minor
  muscles

Modified from Mathers LH et al: *Clinical anatomy principles*, St. Louis, 1996, Mosby
For use in Fritz: *Mosby's Massage Therapy Review*
Copyright © 2002, Mosby, *A Harcourt Health Sciences Company*

Answers are on pages 233–242.

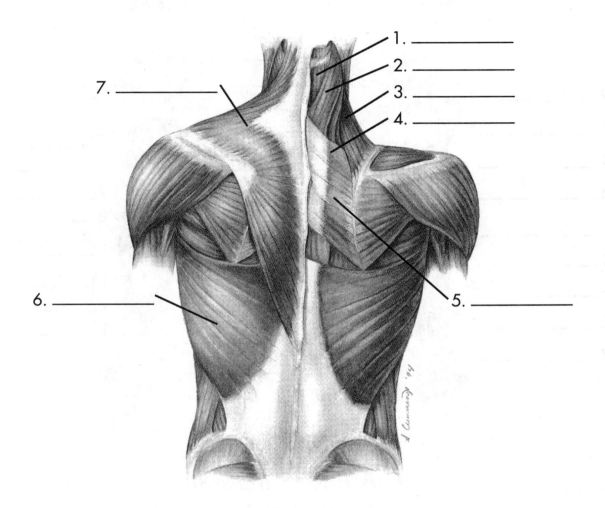

Labeling Exercise 37
Back Muscles: First (Left) and Second (Right) Layers

Choices

Latissimus dorsi muscle   Semispinalis capitis muscle
Levator scapulae muscle   Splenius capitis muscle
Rhomboid major muscle   Trapezius muscle
Rhomboid minor muscle

Modified from Cramer GD, Darby SA: *Basic and clinical anatomy of the spine, spinal cord, and ANS*, St. Louis, 1995, Mosby
For use in Fritz: *Mosby's Massage Therapy Review*
Copyright © 2002, Mosby, *A Harcourt Health Sciences Company*

Answers are on pages 233–242.

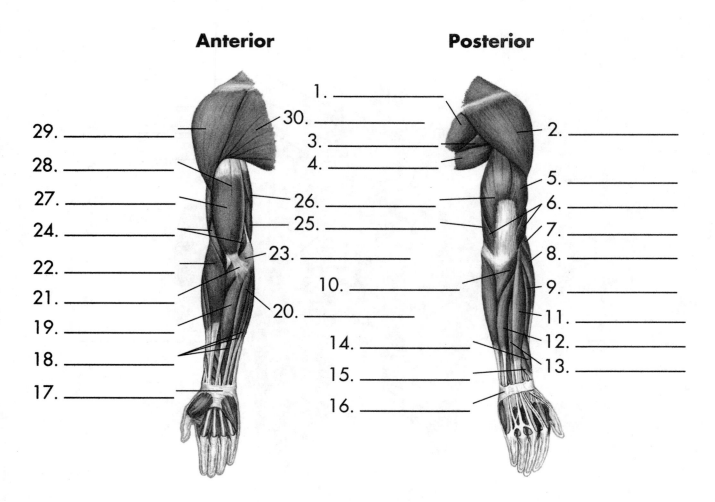

Anterior

Posterior

Labeling Exercise 38
Muscles of Arm

Choices

Abductor pollicis brevis	Extensor carpi radialis brevis	Infraspinatus
Abductor pollicis longus	Extensor carpi radialis longus	Palmaris longus
Anconeus	Extensor carpi ulnaris	Pectoralis major
Biceps brachii long head	Extensor digiti minimi	Pronator teres
Biceps brachii short head	Extensor digitorum communis	Teres major
Bicipital aponeurosis	Extensor retinaculum	Teres minor
Brachialis	Flexor carpi radialis	Triceps, lateral head
Brachioradialis (2 times)	Flexor digitorum superficialis	Triceps, long head
Deltoid (2 times)	Flexor retinaculum	Triceps, medial head (2 times)

Modified from Mourad LA: *Orthopedic disorders*, St. Louis, 1991, Mosby
For use in Fritz: *Mosby's Massage Therapy Review*
Copyright © 2002, Mosby, *A Harcourt Health Sciences Company*

Answers are on pages 233–242.

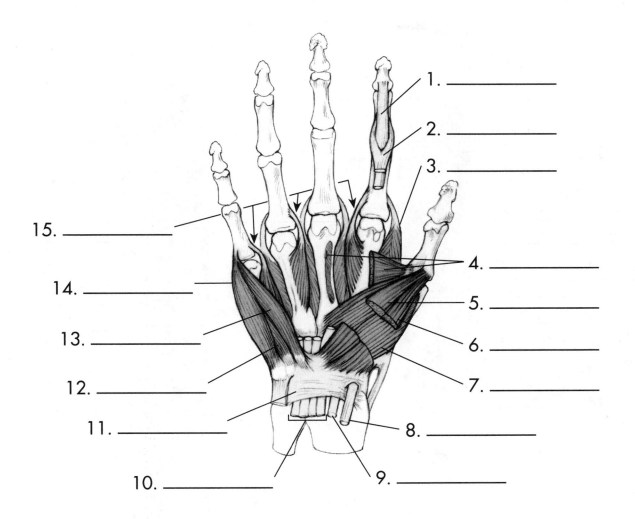

1. _____
2. _____
3. _____
15. _____
14. _____
13. _____
12. _____
11. _____
10. _____
4. _____
5. _____
6. _____
7. _____
8. _____
9. _____

Labeling Exercise 39
Deeper Muscles of Palm: Anterior View

Choices

Abductor digiti minimi muscle
Abductor pollicis brevis muscle
Adductor pollicis muscle
First dorsal interosseous muscle
Flexor digiti minimi muscle
Flexor pollicis brevis muscle
Flexor retinaculum

Opponens digiti minimi muscle
Opponens pollicis muscle
Palmar interossei
Tendon of flexor carpi radialis muscle
Tendon of flexor digitorum profundus

Tendon of flexor digitorum superficialis
Tendon of pollicis longus muscle
Tendons of flexor digitorum superficialis muscle

Modified from Mathers LH et al: *Clinical anatomy principles*, St. Louis, 1996, Mosby
For use in Fritz: *Mosby's Massage Therapy Review*
Copyright © 2002, Mosby, *A Harcourt Health Sciences Company*

Anterior   **Posterior**

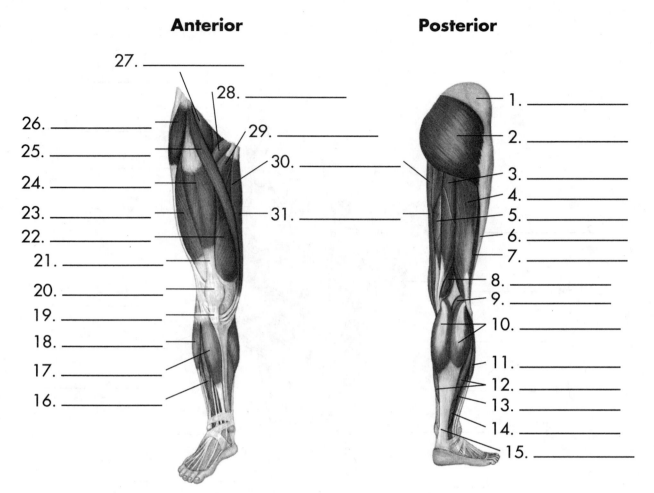

Labeling Exercise 40
Muscles of Leg

Choices

Adductor longus

Adductor magnus

Biceps femoris long head

Biceps femoris short head

Calcaneal tendon (Achilles tendon)

Extensor digitorum longus

Fascia over gluteus medius

Flexor hallucis longus

Gastrocnemius

Gluteus maximus

Gracilis

Iliopsoas

Iliotibial tract

Patella

Patellar ligament

Pectineus

Peroneus brevis

Peroneus longus (2 times)

Plantaris

Rectus femoris

Sartorius

Semimembranosus (2 times)

Semitendinosus

Soleus

Tendon of rectus femoris

Tensor of fasciae latae

Tibialis anterior

Vastus lateralis

Vastus medialis

Modified from Mourad LA: *Orthopedic disorders*, St. Louis, 1991, Mosby
For use in Fritz: *Mosby's Massage Therapy Review*
Copyright © 2002, Mosby, *A Harcourt Health Sciences Company*

Answers are on pages 233–242.

Answer Key for Labeling Exercises

Labeling Exercise 1

1. Rough endoplasmic reticulum
2. Lysosome
3. Golgi apparatus
4. Nucleolus
5. Smooth endoplasmic reticulum
6. Ribosomes
7. Cytoplasm
8. Nucleus
9. Mitochondria
10. Cell (plasma) membrane

Labeling Exercise 2

1. Spinal cord
2. Spinal ganglion
3. Epineurium
4. Perineurium
5. Endoneurium
6. Axon
7. Motor end plate
8. Skin
9. Pain receptors
10. Muscle
11. Myelin sheath
12. Node of Ranvier
13. Nerve bundle (fasciculus)
14. Blood vessels

Labeling Exercise 3

1. Frontal bone
2. Skull
3. Orbit
4. Nasal bone
5. Maxilla
6. Mandible
7. Sternum
8. Ribs
9. Vertebral column
10. Coccyx
11. Zygomatic bone
12. Clavicle
13. Scapula
14. Humerus
15. Coxal (hip) bone
16. Ulna
17. Radius
18. Sacrum
19. Carpals
20. Metacarpals
21. Phalanges
22. Femur
23. Patella
24. Tibia
25. Fibula
26. Tarsals
27. Metatarsals
28. Phalanges
29. Parietal bone
30. Occipital bone
31. Cervical vertebrae
32. Thoracic vertebrae
33. Ribs
34. Lumbar vertebrae
35. Coccyx

Labeling Exercise 4

1. Cervical curve
2. Thoracic curve
3. Lumbar curve
4. Sacral curve
5. First cervical vertebra (atlas)
6. Second cervical vertebra (axis)
7. Seventh cervical vertebra
8. First thoracic vertebra
9. Intervertebral disk
10. Intervertebral foramina
11. First lumbar vertebra
12. Body
13. Transverse process
14. Spinous process

Labeling Exercise 5

1. Jugular notch
2. Seventh cervical vertebra
3. First thoracic vertebra
4. Manubrium
5. Sternal angle
6. Body
7. Xiphoid process
8. Sternum
9. Floating ribs
10. False ribs
11. Costal cartilage
12. True ribs
13. Clavicle
14. Sternal end
15. Body
16. Head
17. Articular facets for body of vertebrae
18. Neck
19. Articular facet for transverse process of vertebra
20. Tubercle
21. Angle
22. Xiphoid process
23. Facets for attachment of costal cartilages 1 to 7
24. Jugular notch
25. Clavicular notch
26. Manubrium
27. Sternal angle
28. Body

Labeling Exercise 6

1. Sternal end
2. Body
3. Acromial end

Labeling Exercise 7

1. Scapular spine
2. Supraspinous fossa
3. Suprascapular notch
4. Infraspinous fossa
5. Infraglenoid tubercle
6. Glenoid fossa
7. Supraglenoid tubercle
8. Acromion
9. Coracoid process
10. Spinoglenoid notch
11. Subscapular fossa
12. Vertebral border
13. Lateral border
14. Scapular spine
15. Coracoid fossa
16. Glenoid fossa

Labeling Exercise 8

1. Greater tubercle
2. Head
3. Greater tubercle
4. Lesser tubercle
5. Anatomic neck
6. Surgical neck
7. Intertubercular groove
8. Deltoid tuberosity
9. Shaft of humerus
10. Radial groove
11. Lateral supracondylar ridge
12. Radial fossa
13. Lateral epicondyle
14. Capitulum
15. Trochlea
16. Coronoid fossa
17. Medial epicondyle
18. Medial epicondylar groove
19. Trochlea
20. Olecranon fossa
21. Medial supracondylar ridge

Labeling Exercise 9
1. Radial head
2. Radial tuberosity
3. Radius
4. Radial styloid
5. Ulnar styloid
6. Ulna
7. Interosseous membrane
8. Trochlear notch
9. Olecranon process of ulna

Labeling Exercise 10
1. Phalanges
2. Metacarpus
3. Carpus
4. Hamate
5. Pisiform
6. Triquetrum
7. Lunate
8. Styloid process
9. Ulnar head
10. Ulna
11. Radius
12. Ulnar notch of radius
13. Styloid process
14. Scaphoid
15. Capitate
16. Trapezium
17. Trapezoid
18. Sesamoids
19. Proximal
20. Middle
21. Distal

Labeling Exercise 11
1. Sacroiliac joint
2. Sacrum
3. Ilium
4. Pubis
5. Ischium
6. Symphysis pubis
7. Obturator foramen
8. Anterior superior iliac spine
9. Sacral promontory
10. Iliac crest
11. Ilium
12. Anterior superior iliac spine
13. Anterior inferior iliac spine
14. Lunate surface
15. Acetabulum
16. Acetabular notch
17. Inferior pubic ramus
18. Ischial ramus
19. Obturator foramen
20. Ischial tuberosity
21. Lesser sciatic notch
22. Ischial spine
23. Greater sciatic notch
24. Posterior inferior iliac spine
25. Posterior superior iliac spine
26. Iliac crest
27. Auricular surface
28. Posterior superior iliac spine
29. Posterior inferior iliac spine
30. Greater sciatic notch
31. Body of ischium
32. Ischial spine
33. Lesser sciatic notch
34. Ischial ramus
35. Inferior pubic ramus
36. Obturator foramen
37. Symphysis pubis
38. Pubic crest
39. Superior pubic ramus
40. Iliopectineal line
41. Anterior inferior iliac spine
42. Anterior superior iliac spine
43. Iliac fossa
44. Ilium

Labeling Exercise 12
1. Greater trochanter
2. Fovea capitis
3. Head of femur
4. Greater trochanter
5. Neck
6. Intertrochanteric fossa
7. Gluteal tuberosity
8. Lesser trochanter
9. Intertrochanteric line
10. Intertrochanteric crest
11. Pectineal line
12. Linea aspera
13. Lateral and medial supracondylar ridges
14. Medial and lateral supracondylar lines
15. Patellar groove
16. Adductor tubercle
17. Lateral epicondyle
18. Medial epicondyle
19. Lateral condyle
20. Medial condyle
21. Intercondylar fossa

Labeling Exercise 13
1. Intercondylar eminence
2. Medial condyle
3. Tibial tuberosity
4. Tibia
5. Medial malleolus
6. Lateral malleolus
7. Fibula
8. Neck of fibula
9. Head
10. Lateral condyle

Labeling Exercise 14
1. Tarsals
2. Lateral cuneiform
3. Cuboid
4. Calcaneus
5. Talus
6. Navicular
7. Tarsals
8. Intermediate cuneiform
9. Medial cuneiform
10. Metatarsals
11. Phalanges
12. Proximal phalanx
13. Middle phalanx
14. Distal phalanx
15. Distal phalanx of great toe
16. Proximal phalanx of great toe
17. Phalanges
18. Metatarsals
19. Tarsals
20. Calcaneus
21. Cuboid
22. Talus
23. Fibula
24. Tibia
25. Talus
26. Navicular
27. Cuneiforms

Labeling Exercise 15
1. Bursa
2. Joint cavity (filled with synovial fluid)
3. Bone
4. Blood vessel
5. Nerve
6. Synovial membrane
7. Fibrous capsule
8. Joint capsule
9. Fibrous layer
10. Membranous layer
11. Periosteum
12. Bone
13. Articular cartilage
14. Tendon sheath

Labeling Exercise 16
1. Coronal suture
2. Sagittal suture
3. Occipital bone
4. Parietal bone
5. Frontal bone

Labeling Exercise 17
1. Condylar process of mandible
2. Articular disk
3. Anterior tubercle, zygoma
4. Lateral temporomandibular ligament
5. Temporal bone, squamous part
6. Sphenoid, greater wing
7. Zygoma
8. Maxilla
9. Mandible
10. Pterygomandibular septae
11. Two heads of lateral pterygoid m.
12. Stylomandibular ligament
13. External auditory meatus

Labeling Exercise 18
1. Humerus
2. Long head of biceps m.
3. Transverse humeral ligament
4. Acromioclavicular ligament
5. Coracoclavicular ligament
6. Conoid ligament
7. Trapezoid ligament
8. Clavicle
9. Transverse scapular ligament
10. Suprascapular notch
11. Glenohumeral ligament
12. Scapula
13. Acromioclavicular ligament
14. Scapular spine and acromion

Labeling Exercise 19
1. Interclavicular ligament
2. Manubrium of sternum
3. Sternoclavicular ligament
4. Clavicle
5. First rib
6. Costoclavicular ligament
7. Second rib
8. Costal cartilages
9. Body of sternum
10. Synovial chondrosternal joint
11. Sternoclavicular joint
12. Articular disk

Labeling Exercise 20
1. Sternum
2. Clavicle
3. Coracoclavicular ligament
4. Acromioclavicular ligament
5. Coracoid process
6. Clavicle
7. Inferior border of scapula
8. Infraspinous fossa
9. Acromion
10. Scapular spine
11. Subscapular fossa

Labeling Exercise 21
1. Lateral epicondyle
2. Medial epicondyle
3. Elbow joint capsule
4. Ulnar collateral ligament
5. Ulna
6. Radius
7. Annular ligament of radius
8. Radial collateral ligament
9. Radial tuberosity
10. Annular ligament
11. Anterior elbow capsule
12. Medial (ulnar) collateral ligament
13. Anterior band
14. Oblique band
15. Posterior band
16. Olecranon of ulna
17. Ulna
18. Radius

Labeling Exercise 22

1. Distal phalanges
2. Middle phalanges
3. Proximal phalanges
4. Metacarpals
5. Hamate
6. Pisiform
7. Triquetrum
8. Capitate
9. Lunate
10. Scaphoid
11. Trapezium
12. Trapezoid
13. Carpometacarpal
14. Metacarpophalangeal
15. Interphalangeal
16. Metacarpophalangeal (MCP)
17. Proximal interphalangeal (PIP)
18. Distal interphalangeal (DIP)

Labeling Exercise 23

1. Iliolumbar ligament
2. Sacroiliac joint
3. Greater sciatic foramen
4. Arcuate line
5. Inguinal ligament
6. Lesser sciatic foramen
7. Acetabulum
8. Coccyx
9. Pubic symphysis
10. Pubic tubercle
11. Pectineal line
12. Sacrotuberous
13. Sacrospinous ligament
14. Sacroiliac ligament

Labeling Exercise 24

1. Ilium
2. Ischiofemoral ligament
3. Greater trochanter
4. Lesser trochanter
5. Ischial tuberosity
6. Inferior pubic ramus
7. Pubofemoral ligament
8. Lesser trochanter
9. Greater trochanter
10. Iliofemoral ligament

Labeling Exercise 25

1. Anterior cruciate ligament
2. Fibular (lateral) collateral ligament
3. Tendon of popliteus muscle
4. Lateral meniscus
5. Transverse ligament
6. Fibular head
7. Patella
8. Patellar ligament
9. Medial meniscus
10. Tibial (medial) collateral ligament
11. Medial condyle
12. Posterior cruciate ligament
13. Posterior meniscus femoral ligament
14. Fibular collateral ligament
15. Lateral condyle
16. Lateral meniscus
17. Popliteus tendon
18. Fibular head
19. Oblique popliteal ligament
20. Tibia
21. Popliteus muscle
22. Semimembranous tendon

Labeling Exercise 26

1. Medial malleolus
2. Anterior tibiotalar
3. Tibionavicular
4. Tibiocalcaneal
5. Posterior tibiotalar
6. Calcaneus
7. Navicular
8. Medial cuneiform

Labeling Exercise 27
1. Fascicle
2. Muscle fiber
3. Myofibril
4. Sarcolemma
5. Nucleus
6. Endomysium
7. Perimysium
8. Epimysium

Labeling Exercise 28
1. Superficial temporal artery
2. Facial artery
3. Common carotid artery
4. Axillary artery
5. Brachial artery
6. Radial artery
7. Femoral artery
8. Popliteal artery
9. Dorsalis pedis artery

Labeling Exercise 29
1. Tonsils
2. Cervical lymph node
3. Entrance of thoracic duct into subclavian vein
4. Axillary lymph node
5. Mammary plexus
6. Spleen
7. Peyer's patches in intestinal wall
8. Inguinal lymph nodes
9. Bone marrow
10. Appendix
11. Intestinal lymph nodes
12. Thoracic duct
13. Right lymphatic duct
14. Thymus gland

Labeling Exercise 30
1. Pharynx
2. Trachea
3. Left main bronchus
4. Alveolus
5. Alveolar sac
6. Alveolar duct
7. Pleural space
8. Pleura
9. Bronchiole
10. Right main bronchus

Labeling Exercise 31
1. Urinary bladder
2. Symphysis pubis
3. Prostate gland
4. Corpus cavernosum
5. Corpus spongiosum
6. Urethra
7. Testis
8. Glans
9. Bulbocavernosus muscle
10. Anus
11. Ejaculatory duct
12. Levator ani muscle
13. Seminal vesicle
14. Rectum

Labeling Exercise 32
1. Rectouterine fossa
2. Oviduct
3. Ovary
4. Uterus
5. Vesicouterine fossa
6. Bladder
7. Pubic symphysis
8. Clitoris
9. Urethral orifice
10. Vagina
11. Vaginal introitus
12. Labium minus
13. Urogenital diaphragm
14. Perineal body
15. Anal orifice
16. Anococcygeal raphe
17. Coccyx

Labeling Exercise 33
1. Cerebrum
2. Cerebellum
3. Brachial plexus
4. Musculocutaneous nerve
5. Spinal cord
6. Saphenous nerve
7. Digital nerves
8. Perineal nerve
9. Tibial nerve
10. Femoral cutaneous nerve
11. Ischial nerve
12. Femoral nerve
13. Cauda equina
14. Intercostal nerves

Labeling Exercise 34
1. Facial muscles
2. Cranial muscles
3. Sternocleidomastoideus
4. Trapezius
5. Pectoralis major
6. Serratus anterior
7. Rectus abdominis
8. Flexors of wrist and fingers
9. Obliquus externus
10. Tensor fasciae latae
11. Vastus lateralis
12. Rectus femoris
13. Patella
14. Tibialis anterior
15. Extensor digitorum longus
16. Peroneus longus
17. Peroneus brevis
18. Extensor hallucis longus tendon
19. Superior extensor retinaculum
20. Soleus
21. Gastrocnemius
22. Patellar tendon
23. Vastus medialis
24. Sartorius
25. Flexor retinaculum
26. Adductors of thigh
27. Extensors of wrist and fingers
28. Linea alba
29. Biceps brachii

30. Deltoideus

Labeling Exercise 35
1. Splenius capitis
2. Trapezius
3. Infraspinatus
4. Portion of rhomboideus
5. Obliquus externus
6. Gluteus maximus
7. Adductor magnus
8. Gracilis
9. Iliotibial tract
10. Plantaris
11. Gastrocnemius tendon (Achilles tendon)
12. Soleus
13. Superior peroneal retinaculum
14. Peroneus brevis
15. Peroneus longus
16. Gastrocnemius
17. Semimembranosus
18. Biceps femoris
19. Semitendinosus
20. Extensors of the wrist and fingers
21. Latissimus dorsi
22. Triceps
23. Teres major
24. Teres minor
25. Deltoideus
26. Seventh cervical vertebra
27. Sternocleidomastoideus

Labeling Exercise 36
1. Frontalis muscle
2. Temporalis muscle
3. Procerus muscle
4. Orbicularis oculi m. (palpebral part)
5. Levator labii superioris
6. Zygomaticus major and minor muscles
7. Levator anguli oris
8. Parotid gland and duct
9. Buccinator muscle
10. Masseter muscle
11. Orbicularis oris muscle
12. Depressor labii inferioris
13. Mentalis
14. Depressor anguli oris
15. Platysma
16. Risorius
17. Nasalis
18. Zygomaticus major muscle
19. Zygomaticus minor muscle
20. Levator labii superioris alaeque nasi muscle
21. Orbicularis oculi (orbital part)
22. Frontalis muscle
23. Temporalis muscle
24. Procerus muscle
25. Orbicularis oculi muscle
26. Levator labii superioris alaeque nasi muscle
27. Nasalis muscle
28. Zygomaticus minor muscle
29. Zygomaticus major muscle
30. Orbicularis oris muscle
31. Depressor labii inferioris
32. Depressor anguli oris muscle
33. Mentalis muscle
34. Platysma muscle
35. Buccinator muscle
36. Masseter muscle
37. Parotid gland and duct
38. Auricular muscles
39. Superior
40. Posterior
41. Anterior
42. Occipitalis muscle
43. Galea aponeurotica

Labeling Exercise 37
1. Semispinalis capitis muscle
2. Splenius capitis muscle
3. Levator scapulae muscle
4. Rhomboid minor muscle
5. Rhomboid major muscle
6. Latissimus dorsi muscle
7. Trapezius muscle

Labeling Exercise 38
1. Infraspinatus
2. Deltoid
3. Teres minor
4. Teres major
5. Triceps, long head
6. Triceps, medial head
7. Brachioradialis
8. Extensor carpi radialis longus
9. Extensor carpi radialis brevis
10. Anconeus
11. Extensor digitorum communis
12. Extensor carpi ulnaris
13. Extensor digiti minimi
14. Abductor pollicis brevis
15. Abductor pollicis longus
16. Extensor retinaculum
17. Flexor retinaculum
18. Flexor digitorum superficialis
19. Flexor carpi radialis
20. Palmaris longus
21. Bicipital aponeurosis
22. Brachioradialis
23. Pronator teres
24. Brachialis
25. Triceps, medial head
26. Triceps, lateral head
27. Biceps brachii, long head
28. Biceps brachii, short head
29. Deltoid
30. Pectoralis major

Labeling Exercise 39

1. Tendon of flexor digitorum profundus
2. Tendon of flexor digitorum superficialis
3. First dorsal interosseous muscle
4. Adductor pollicis muscle
5. Flexor pollicis brevis muscle
6. Abductor pollicis brevis muscle
7. Opponens pollicis muscle
8. Tendon of flexor carpi radialis muscle
9. Tendon of pollicis longus muscle
10. Tendons of flexor digitorum superficialis muscle
11. Flexor retinaculum
12. Opponens digiti minimi muscle
13. Flexor digiti minimi muscle
14. Abductor digiti minimi muscle
15. Palmar interossei

Labeling Exercise 40

1. Fascia over gluteus medius
2. Gluteus maximus
3. Semitendinosus
4. Biceps femoris long head
5. Semimembranosus
6. Iliotibial tract
7. Biceps femoris short head
8. Semimembranosus
9. Plantaris
10. Gastrocnemius
11. Peroneus longus
12. Soleus
13. Peroneus brevis
14. Flexor hallucis longus
15. Calcaneal tendon (Achilles tendon)
16. Extensor digitorum longus
17. Tibialis anterior
18. Peroneus longus
19. Patellar ligament
20. Patella
21. Tendon of rectus femoris
22. Vastus medialis
23. Vastus lateralis
24. Rectus femoris
25. Sartorius
26. Tensor of fasciae latae
27. Iliopsoas
28. Pectineus
29. Adductor longus
30. Adductor magnus
31. Gracilis

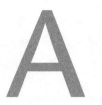

Practice Test One

1. *Which of the following is a quantified outcome goal?*

   a. Client will be able to increase range of motion of the lateral flexion of the cervical area by 15 degrees
   b. Client will be able to resume normal work activities
   c. Client will be reassessed in 12 sessions
   d. Client will recover ability to play golf

2. *Condition management involves the use of massage methods to support clients who cannot undergo a therapeutic change who but wish to be as effective as possible within an existing set of circumstances. Which of the following is an example of condition management?*

   a. Managing the existing physical compensation patterns
   b. Assisting the client through learning to walk again
   c. Restoring a client's range of motion to preinjury state
   d. Using massage to help a client feel better about self and to change jobs

3. *Nerve impingement syndromes occur primarily in plexus areas. A person experiencing an impingement in the cervical plexus would have _____.*

   a. Shoulder pain, chest pain, arm pain, wrist pain, and hand pain
   b. Low-back discomfort with a belt distribution of pain as well as pain in lower abdomen, genitals, and thigh
   c. Gluteal pain, leg pain, genital pain, and foot pain
   d. Headaches, neck pain, and breathing difficulties

4. *Which of the following is **not** a general benefit of massage?*

   a. Improvement in circulation
   b. Enhanced elimination
   c. Inhibition of homeostasis
   d. Increased levels of endorphins

5. *The most effective massage methods to work on impingement syndromes are _____.*

   a. Tapotement and shaking
   b. Muscle energy and lengthening
   c. Rapid deep compression
   d. Friction

6. *The origin of pain can be somatic or visceral. Somatic pain is defined as _____.*

   a. Pain from only stimulation of receptors in the skin
   b. Pain from only stimulation of receptors in the skeletal muscles, joints, or tendons
   c. Pain resulting from only stimulation of receptors in the internal organs
   d. Pain arising from stimulation of receptors in the skin, skeletal muscles, joints, tendons, and fascia

7. *The simplest, most effective deterrent to the spread of disease is _____.*

   a. Handwashing
   b. Sterilization technique
   c. Using a towel barrier
   d. Keeping shots up-to-date

8. *The inflammatory response can occur to any tissue injury. This response has four signs: redness, swelling, pain, and _____.*

   a. Stickiness
   b. Liquid
   c. Heat
   d. Mucus

                    Answers are on page 295.

9. *You are running behind today and your next client has been waiting for 15 minutes. It is most important that you _____.*

    a. Maintain your scheduled appointments on time
    b. Have materials and activities available for clients to entertain themselves
    c. Make sure sheets and linens are changed and equipment disinfected between massages
    d. Apologize to the client for being late

10. *A client keeps complaining of discomfort at the end of the massage stroke. What is happening?*

    a. The practitioner is pushing with the legs
    b. The practitioner is off balance and using counterpressure
    c. The skin is being pulled from lack of lubricant
    d. The compressive force is distributed over a narrow base at the end of the stroke

11. *When stretching the legs of a client by applying a pull against the ankle, the massage practitioner should _____.*

    a. Fix the feet and pull with the shoulders
    b. Move to a symmetrical stance and lean back
    c. Maintain asymmetrical stance, lean back, keeping the back straight
    d. Bend the knees and push back

12. *Which of the following is **not** a safe professional practice?*

    a. Assisting the elderly on and off the massage table
    b. Burning candles for atmosphere in the massage room
    c. Maintaining good lighting in massage areas
    d. Regularly checking cables of portable massage tables

13. *To prevent allergic reactions, all lubricant should be _____.*

    a. Oil based
    b. Water based
    c. Dispensed in sanitary fashion
    d. Scent free

14. *A massage professional wants to check to see if the location for an office being considered for rental is in an appropriate business distinct. Where does one find this information?*

    a. Local zoning office
    b. Facility rental agreement
    c. State licensing bureau
    d. County clerk's office

15. *When a practitioner is in a relaxed standing posture supporting the gravitational line with the normal knee-locked position, which muscles are used for balance?*

    a. Psoas
    b. Gastrocnemius
    c. Hamstrings
    d. Quadriceps

16. *When one is applying compressive force down and forward, weight is most efficient if kept _____.*

    a. On the back leg and foot
    b. On the front leg and knee
    c. On the back foot and toes
    d. On the front foot and toes

17. *A massage practitioner has been experiencing increasingly severe low-back pain. The practice is full time with 20 clients per week. What could the massage practitioner do to reduce back strain?*

    a. Bend the knees while performing massage
    b. Raise the table height to prevent torso bending
    c. Keep the head forward and down to change the center of gravity
    d. Externally rotate the back foot away from the line of force

18. *A massage professional is feeling strain in the knees. Which of the following is the most logical cause?*

    a. Doing massage on hard floors
    b. Working with clients in the side-lying position
    c. Keeping the knees flexed and static
    d. Moving whenever the arm reach is beyond 60 degrees

                    Answers are on page 295.

19. *The most important stability feature of a portable massage table is _____.*

    a. Frame
    b. Cable support
    c. Adjustable legs
    d. Center hinge

20. *Regardless of the type of draping material used, which of the following is required?*

    a. Disposable
    b. Large
    c. Opaque
    d. Cotton fabric

21. *A massage professional has just rented office space and fully decorated the area. There is a window in the massage room and both overhead and indirect lighting. There is a central thermostat in another area, but the massage room has both a fan and an electric heater to adjust temperature. The small waiting area is bright and comfortable, with many sorts of flowering plants. There is a private restroom just off the waiting room. The massage room does not have a closet but does have hooks for the clients' clothing. A closed cabinet holds supplies. The business area is small but has a locked file cabinet and small desk. What suggestion would you make for improving the massage environment?*

    a. Add an aromatherapy atomizer
    b. Put a lock on the massage room door
    c. Move the file cabinet into the massage room
    d. Remove the flowering plants

22. *A massage practitioner has been seeing the same client weekly for 3 months. The client often discusses personal issues with the massage practitioner. Last session the massage professional provided some reading information to help the client and talked with the client about how the practitioner had dealt with a similar issue. The client has canceled the last two appointments. What is the most logical cause?*

    a. Feedback about the massage broke down
    b. Conversation with the client overshadowed the massage session
    c. Gender issues are influencing the session
    d. The orientation process needs to be repeated

23. *A client complains of a mild general low back pain. Which of the following is appropriate?*

    a. Use side-lying position with knee support
    b. Work with client prone, using support under abdomen and ankles
    c. Work with client supine, using support only under the neck
    d. Position client in seated position and avoid supports

24. *Massage has been shown to slow formation of scar tissue and helps keep scar tissue pliable. This assists the healing process by _____.*

    a. Blocking the action of antihistamines
    b. Counterbalancing the defect in the body
    c. Promoting regeneration and keeping replacement to a minimum
    d. Keeping the functioning energy reserves in place

25. *In which situation would you stay in the massage room and assist a client on and off the massage table?*

    a. A client in the first trimester of pregnancy
    b. A 65-year-old male with diabetes
    c. An elderly female with high blood pressure
    d. An adolescent with a wrist cast

                    Answers are on page 295.

26. Massage manipulations are _____.

   a. Skillful use of the hands and forearms to directly affect the soft tissue
   b. Skillful use of the hands to directly affect the joints
   c. Application of methods using heat and equipment to affect soft tissue
   d. Application of compressive forces to affect meridians

27. A client has an outcome goal for the massage of increased circulation and range of motion for the knee. Which of the following is the best approach?

   a. Reflexive methods focused on chemical changes
   b. Mechanical methods focused on the area
   c. Mechanical methods to reflexively influence neuroactivity
   d. Reflexive methods to increase compressive force to the viscera

28. Which of the following methods is most beneficial for abdominal massage to mechanically encourage fecal movement in the large intestine?

   a. Effleurage
   b. Resting position
   c. Tapotement
   d. Compression

29. A client reports a sensitivity to lubricant during the history and would like a massage in which no lubricant is used. Which method would be **inappropriate?**

   a. Shaking
   b. Compression
   c. Kneading
   d. Effleurage

30. A client complains of restricted range of motion in the shoulder. The primary outcome for the massage is to increase shoulder mobility. Which method would be the best choice?

   a. Friction
   b. Muscle energy
   c. Hydrotherapy
   d. Resting stroke

31. Which of the following methods would be best for assessing for the physiologic and pathologic motion barrier?

   a. Passive joint movement
   b. Active resistive movement
   c. Postisometric relaxation
   d. Concentric isotonic contraction

32. The definition of health is _____.

   a. Prepathologic state
   b. Homeostatic and restorative body mechanisms can no longer adapt
   c. Anatomic and physiologic functioning limits
   d. Optimal functioning with freedom from disease or abnormal processes

33. Which component is essential for effective application of joint movement?

   a. Stabilization to isolate the movement to the targeted joint
   b. Tapotement to stimulate the joint kinesthetic receptors
   c. High-velocity manipulative movement
   d. Cross-directional tissue stretching to cause traction on the joint capsule

34. A client is feeling fatigued and does not wish to participate during the massage. Instead the client wishes to remain passive and quiet. Which of the following muscle energy methods would be appropriate?

   a. Positional release
   b. Pulsed muscle energy
   c. Integrated approach
   d. Approximation

                    Answers are on page 295.

35. A client has been receiving massage weekly for 2 months. The main goal for the massage is increased mobility in the lumbar and hip region. The client has experienced stiffness and reduced ability since a fall off a bike 2 years ago. General massage and muscle energy methods with lengthening have produced mild improvement. Which of the following mechanical methods has the potential to increase results?

    a. Lymphatic drainage
    b. Stretching
    c. Contract/relax
    d. Strain-counterstrain

36. A client is requesting extensive massage to the neck and upper shoulders. Which is the most efficient client position to easily massage these areas?

    a. Prone
    b. Supine
    c. Seated
    d. Side-lying

37. A client complains of a stiff and stuck feeling in the lumbar area. Assessment indicates that the fascia in that area is thick and adhered to the underlying tissue. Which method would best restore pliability to this tissue?

    a. Skin rolling
    b. Shaking
    c. Friction
    d. Vibration
    d. Right thigh extensors

38. A major contraindication to massage of the legs is _____.

    a. Acne
    b. Brachial nerve compression
    c. Disk compression
    d. Thrombophlebitis

39. Which of the following methods is best for general broad applications when lubricant is requested?

    a. Petrissage
    b. Compression
    c. Effleurage
    d. Vibration

40. A client is complaining about pain and stiffness in the neck but is particularly sensitive to pressure used in the neck area, flinching and stiffening in a protective stance whenever the neck is massaged. The current approach is to primarily use petrissage with the client in the prone position. What is the best alternative?

    a. Change position to supine and use effleurage
    b. Use side-lying position and broad-based compression
    c. Combine passive range of motion, muscle energy, and friction with client seated
    d. Have client seated and then use deep petrissage

41. After tripping down a stair, but not falling, a client describes a sudden onset of pain during twisting and reaching movements. Which type of biomechanical dysfunction is most likely to be occurring?

    a. Neuromuscular
    b. Myofascial
    c. Joint related
    d. Capsular pattern

42. Which of the following body areas is often massaged longer than is effective?

    a. Hands
    b. Abdomen
    c. Legs
    d. Back

 Answers are on page 295.

43. A client has been receiving massage for a mild peripheral arterial circulation problem. Which of the following would be an appropriate self-help method to teach the client?

   a. Lymphatic drainage
   b. Skin rolling
   c. Alternating applications of hot and cold
   d. Frictioning

44. The secondary effect of a local cold application is _____.

   a. Sedative
   b. Increased localized circulation
   c. Diaphoretic
   d. Decreased systemic circulation

45. A folded towel soaked in water of the desired temperature and placed on a large area of skin is called a _____.

   a. Tonic friction
   b. Vaporizer
   c. Sponge
   d. Pack

46. A massage client reports that after the massage she had some itchy areas of skin. Her clothes felt rough against her skin. Which neurotransmitter may be involved?

   a. Histamine
   b. Acetylcholine
   c. Epinephrine
   d. CCK

47. A client has mild edema in her lower legs from a long plane flight the previous day. Which of the following is an appropriate treatment plan?

   a. Short light gliding strokes focused on the legs. Compression to the soles of the feet. Active and passive joint movement for the ankle, knee, and hip. Placing the legs above the heart.
   b. Compression to the legs focused on the medial side from proximal to distal. Muscle energy and lengthening combined with stretching in the area of the most accumulation of fluid.
   c. Deep gliding strokes from proximal to distal on the legs. Placing the legs above the heart. Limiting movement to encourage drainage.
   d. Superficial and deep compression along the vessels in the lateral leg. Active resistive joint movement combined with shaking.

48. Because of a skin condition, general massage is contraindicated for a client, but he is allowed to have his feet and hands worked on. He complains of neck stiffness. If using foot reflexology theory, where would the massage practitioner focus massage on the foot to affect the neck?

   a. Heel
   b. Tips of the toes
   c. Base of the large toe
   d. Sole of the foot

49. Therapeutic inflammation is best utilized in situations _____.

   a. In which there is a compromised immune function
   b. Resolving a fibrotic connective tissue dysfunction
   c. In which active inflammation is already present
   d. In which a condition like fibromyalgia exists

          Answers are on page 295.

50. *A client injured his right shoulder 3 years ago. Assessment indicates decreased mobility of the skin surrounding the shoulder coupled with a painful but normal range of motion. Which is the best treatment option for this client?*

    a. Deep transverse friction
    b. Superficial myofascial release
    c. Compression
    d. Lymphatic drainage

51. *Deep transverse friction applied correctly will _____.*

    a. Inhibit circulation
    b. Create controlled inflammation
    c. Provide broad-based application
    d. Replace broadening contractions

52. *An active trigger point that is left untreated for 6 months often will _____.*

    a. Become an ashi point
    b. Become hot to the touch
    c. Have fibrotic changes
    d. Only elicit referred pain

53. *When treating trigger points, _____.*

    a. Direct pressure methods and squeeze methods should be used first
    b. Positional release with lengthening is the first application method
    c. Connective tissue stretching needs to accompany muscle energy application
    d. Lengthening of the tissue housing the trigger point is only effective with a local tissue stretch

54. *A client is complaining of difficulty hitting a golf ball and describes a sense of timing being off. This could be a result of a disruption in what type of reflex?*

    a. Conditioned reflex
    b. Tendon reflex
    c. Stretch reflex
    d. Mono reflex

55. *In Shiatsu a Ki energy flow that is under energy is called _____.*

    a. Tao
    b. Kyo
    c. Jitsu
    d. AhShi

56. *Which of the following meridians is yin?*

    a. Gallbladder
    b. Stomach
    c. Lung
    d. Large intestine

57. *Which of the following meridians is most medial?*

    a. Central
    b. Spleen
    c. Liver
    d. Large intestine

58. *Which is a correct way to sedate a hyperactive acupuncture point?*

    a. Tap the point
    b. Vibrate the point
    c. Place sustained pressure on the point
    d. Stimulate the meridian containing the point

59. *Going clockwise on the five-element wheel, which element is adjacent to the fire element?*

    a. Earth
    b. Metal
    c. Water
    d. Wood

60. *A client has a cough and nasal mucus, diarrhea, and intestinal cramping. The large intestine meridian is tender to the touch. Which other meridian that is part of the metal element is directly involved?*

    a. Pericardium
    b. Lung
    c. Bladder
    d. Heart

Answers are on page 295.

61. Which of the following is considered an Ayurvedic dosha?

   a. Pitta
   b. Marma
   c. Governing
   d. Ch'I

62. A dosha is physiologically a/n _____.

   a. Nerve pathway
   b. Chemical pattern
   c. Electrical pattern
   d. Dietary pattern

63. In Ayurveda, the chakras are considered _____.

   a. Seven centers of prana located in the aura
   b. Seven centers of ki located on the central meridian
   c. Seven centers of prana located along the spinal column
   d. Six locations of kyo corresponding to centers of consciousness

64. A system that combines the theory of Oriental medicine and Ayurveda is _____.

   a. Polarity
   b. Rolfing
   c. Shiatsu
   d. Reflexology

65. In polarity theory, the left side of the body is considered _____.

   a. Ether
   b. Negative
   c. Neutral
   d. Positive

66. In polarity theory, the color green is associated with which body current?

   a. Ether
   b. Air
   c. Fire
   d. Water

67. In polarity therapy, the joints are considered _____.

   a. Chakra areas
   b. Serpentine brain wave currents
   c. Neutral
   d. Negative

68. During the massage a client often speaks of problems with his children respecting house rules. This is a _____.

   a. Body issue
   b. Mind issue
   c. Spiritual issue
   d. Core issue

69. Wellness programs usually include methods to improve communication. Which of the following best explains why communication is more difficult to improve than diet?

   a. Diet and nutrition are more concrete and objective than subjective communication
   b. Diet is much more dependent on others while communication is independent of others
   c. Stress focuses change toward healthy food choices
   d. Communication skills are highly genetically influenced but diet is not

70. When breathing in the normal relaxed pattern, _____.

   a. The inhale is longer than the exhale
   b. Deep inspiration is accentuated
   c. Accessory muscles only work on exhalation
   d. The exhale is longer than the inhale

71. A client feels fatigued all the time. She explains that she doesn't seem to sleep all night. Which of the following may improve her situation?

   a. An afternoon cup of coffee
   b. Taking a long nap in the afternoon
   c. Going to bed and watching television
   d. Spending at least 30 minutes outdoors

Copyright ©2002 by Mosby, Inc. All rights reserved.

Answers are on page 295.

72. *A client is in the exhaustion phase of the general adaptation response. When one is considering a treatment plan for massage, which of the following is **not** appropriate?*

    a. Ability of the client to expend energy for active change
    b. The availability of support and resources during change process
    c. Practitioner must have appropriate knowledge and skills
    d. Completing outcomes in ten sessions or less

73. *Science is defined as _____.*

    a. Knowing something without going through a conscious process of thinking
    b. The ability to pay attention to a specific area and maintain an unconscious focus and intent
    c. The intellectual process of using all mental and physical resources available to better understand, explain, and predict normal and unusual natural phenomena
    d. Craft, skill, and technique that enable a person to monitor and adjust involuntary or subconscious responses

74. *The techniques of therapeutic massage provide manual external sensory stimulation. Which of the following would be a good example?*

    a. Entrainment
    b. Rubbing
    c. Centering
    d. Breathing

75. *Connectedness and intimacy in massage are most likely the results of an increased level of _____.*

    a. Cortisol
    b. Endorphins
    c. Serotonin
    d. Oxytocin

76. *A client states a goal of wanting to relax and complains of having headaches, gastrointestinal problems, and high blood pressure. The client is likely to be experiencing _____.*

    a. An excessive parasympathetic output
    b. An excessive sympathetic output
    c. An entrainment process normalization
    d. Sleep deprivation

77. *A person experiencing fluid retention, muscle weakness, vertigo, hypersensitivity, fatigue, weight gain, and breakdown in connective tissue most likely has _____.*

    a. Test anxiety
    b. Long-term high blood levels of cortisol
    c. First-stage/alarm reaction
    d. Conservation withdrawal

78. *What type of massage has been demonstrated to be most helpful for a client who has reached the exhaustive reaction phase of stress and been there for over 6 months?*

    a. Several appointments over 1 month using 15 minutes of tapotement and shaking
    b. A massage using pulling and pressing with light pressure for weekly sessions for 3 months
    c. A massage that primarily focuses on long slow strokes, broad-based compression, and rocking for weekly appointments for 6 months
    d. A staccato, fast deep pressure during weekly massage for 6 months

79. *Parasympathetic patterns are _____.*

    a. Restorative—adrenaline is secreted, mobility is decreased, and the bronchioles are constricted
    b. Physical activity is curtailed, digestion and elimination are increased, and the bronchioles are constricted
    c. Physical activity is increased, pupils are dilated, saliva secretion is stopped, and stomach secretion is increased
    d. Restorative—heartbeat speeds up, bladder delays emptying, and saliva secretion increases

  Answers are on page 295.

80. A massage practitioner identifies an area of restricted tissue and immediately uses skin rolling to increase connective tissue pliability. How did this interfere with assessment processes?

    a. The localized treatment did not prove effective
    b. The pattern was changed before it was understood
    c. The therapist did not chart the area prior to the massage
    d. The method was not appropriate to the condition

81. A client becomes very relaxed in response to the music and the rhythm of the strokes used during the massage session. What has occurred?

    a. Mechanical effects
    b. Circulation decrease
    c. Entrainment
    d. Client education

82. There are three main types of proprioceptors: muscle spindles, tendon organs, and _____.

    a. Cervical/lumbar plexus
    b. Spinal nerves
    c. Joint kinesthetic receptors
    d. Sphincter muscles

83. The most common bodywork technique that involves the tendon reflex is _____.

    a. Muscle toning
    b. Postisometric relaxation
    c. Acupuncture
    d. Counterirritation

84. The gallbladder 30 acupuncture point location correlates with which of the following motor points?

    a. Triceps
    b. Gastrocnemius
    c. Gluteus maximus
    d. Brachioradialis

85. The complementary relationship of opposites is described by _____.

    a. Organ and system organization
    b. Responsiveness and metabolism
    c. Yin and yang
    d. Qi and shen

86. The Oriental healing theory of the Law of Five Elements relates best to _____.

    a. Muscle tissue structures
    b. Nervous tissue structures
    c. Organs
    d. Prana

87. A massage professional is considering a position at a local day spa. The owner of the business offered either an employee position at a salary or a subcontractor position based on commission. Which would be an advantage of the employee position?

    a. Variable income
    b. Stable income
    c. Subject to employer's regulations
    d. Independent ability to set work hours

88. Expenses used to begin new business operations are called _____.

    a. Business plan
    b. Reimbursement
    c. Investments
    d. Start-up costs

89. A massage practitioner has just redesigned his brochure and has included the types of massage provided, what the massage is like, information about the practitioners' qualifications, and client responsibilities. What did he forget?

    a. Tax structures
    b. Type of premise liability insurance
    c. Fees
    d. Client-practitioner agreement

 Answers are on page 295.

90. *The type of insurance needed to protect in case a client falls while in the business location is* _____.

   a. Malpractice
   b. Premise liability
   c. Independent contractor liability
   d. Disability

91. *A massage professional becomes angry with a client who complains about personal problems during the massage. The massage practitioner is displaying* _____.

   a. Transference
   b. Therapeutic relationship
   c. Ethical behavior
   d. Countertransference

92. *A massage professional works with three main populations: athletes, those with chronic pain, and clients requiring stress management. The therapist uses a variety of methods. Which of the following best describes the massage application style being used?*

   a. Structural and postural approaches
   b. Applied kinesiology
   c. Integrated approaches
   d. Myofascial methods

93. *A massage professional with entry-level training has been seeing a client recently diagnosed with diabetes. The massage professional is becoming more uncomfortable providing massage as the client displays more symptoms. What is occurring?*

   a. The massage professional is in a dual role now that the client is ill
   b. The client is more demanding of the professional
   c. The massage professional has failed to abide by the definition of massage
   d. The massage professional is functioning outside the personal scope of practice

94. *Which of the following would be an appropriate disclosure to a client?*

   a. The fact that the massage professional has a cold
   b. Business financial concerns
   c. Discussion about a mutual acquaintance
   d. Marital difficulties

95. *A massage professional with 15 years of experience but minimal continuing education is in charge of a massage clinic. A recent massage graduate has obtained a position at the clinic. The new graduate notices that his current skills, particularly in charting and critical thinking, are more sophisticated than those of his supervisor but is hesitant to discuss the issue. What is the best description for this situation?*

   a. Power differential
   b. Dual role
   c. Maintenance of professional environment
   d. Reciprocity

96. *Which of the following would be the best explanation for a client who is confused over an incident of becoming mildly sexually aware during the last massage?*

   a. The massage practitioner was sexualizing the massage
   b. The client was sexualizing the massage
   c. The client was experiencing parasympathetic sensations
   d. The massage practitioner was massaging erotic zones

                                 Answers are on page 295.

97. A client complains of both a congested nose and low back stiffness. What is the logical connection between the two?

    a. The respiratory mucus is too thin and allows bacteria to enter the body, causing a kidney infection
    b. The swell bodies in the nose are not able to function properly, so the normal movement during sleep is disrupted
    c. The olfactory nerves are increasing parasympathetic arousal, causing an increase in muscle tension
    d. Nasal congestion is blocking the sinus cavities and inner ear, changing muscle tone in the lower extremities

98. During assessment a client is observed with mild tachypnea, tension in the muscles of the neck and shoulder, and nervousness. Which of the following is most true?

    a. Nitrogen levels have risen and oxygen levels have decreased, creating a decrease in tidal volume
    b. Oxyhemoglobin is saturated with carbon dioxide and the muscles display tetany
    c. An increase in carbon dioxide in the blood is triggering sympathetic activation
    d. Oxygen levels have increased and carbon dioxide levels have dropped, predisposing to hyperventilation syndrome

99. Massage methods that modulate the breathing rhythm also _____.

    a. Predispose a person to pulmonary embolism
    b. Interfere with treatment for sleep apnea
    c. Interact with the autonomic nervous system
    d. Interfere with most meditation methods

100. Which portion of the small intestine contains ducts from the liver, gallbladder, and pancreas?

    a. Ileum
    b. Jejunum
    c. Duodenum
    d. Mesentery

101. A major function of the large intestine is to _____.

    a. Absorb water
    b. Concentrate bile
    c. Remove and store glycogen
    d. Convert amino acids

102. A regular client reports various digestive upsets including dry mouth and constipation. The physician who wants a treatment plan and justification has cleared the client for massage. Which of the following would be the best plan to submit to the physician?

    a. Stimulating massage coupled with teaching self-help breathing supporting an increase in oxygen and a decrease in carbon dioxide to support ongoing ANS sympathetic dominance
    b. General massage combined with deep massage to the colon to suppress peristalsis and break down concentrated fecal matter
    c. General massage focused to generate relaxation with diaphragmatic breathing and rhythmic stroking to the colon to stimulate peristalsis
    d. General massage to create parasympathetic dominance and lymphatic drainage, with visceral massage to the liver to increase detoxification and support upper chest breathing

103. Which of the following pathologic conditions is considered a medical emergency and requires immediate referral?

    a. Gastroenteritis
    b. Peptic ulcer disease
    c. Inflammatory bowel disease
    d. Strangulated hernia

104. Cystitis is _____.

    a. Inflammation of the medulla of the kidney
    b. Infection of the glomerulus
    c. Bladder infection
    d. Obstruction of the urethra

                    Answers are on page 295.

105. Thirty minutes into a relaxation massage a male client has an erection. What is the most logical reason for this response?

   a. The client has been "sexualizing" the massage

   b. Erection is a parasympathetic response

   c. Stimulation of the skin shifts blood flow

   d. Activation of sympathetic reflexes triggers the response

106. During sexual development in the female, which occurs last?

   a. Hypothalamus matures

   b. Estradiol is produced

   c. Adrenal cortex hormone signals pubic hair growth

   d. Ovulation

107. If a female client is in the second trimester of a pregnancy, which of the following would most apply?

   a. Massage will be most comfortable if it is given with the client prone

   b. Massage will be most comfortable if client is positioned on their side

   c. Massage of the feet is contraindicated

   d. Massage should focus most on lymphatic drainage

108. During massage a lactating client experiences the letdown response. What would be the most likely cause?

   a. Massage stimulates the release of oxytocin

   b. Massage stimulates the production of testosterone

   c. Massage decreases colostrum

   d. Massage decreases libido

109. Which phase of nerve signal conduction is related to muscle energy methods of massage that use some sort of muscle contraction to prepare the muscle to relax and lengthen?

   a. Action potential

   b. Refractory period

   c. Depolarization

   d. Saltatory conduction

110. A client reports before the massage that his mind is agitated. He feels like he wants to scream. He is talking loudly and pacing. After the massage he feels calmer and wants a nap. Which neurotransmitter is largely responsible for the mood change?

   a. Norepinephrine

   b. Dopamine

   c. Serotonin

   d. Substance P

111. Why do the primary motor and the primary somesthetic sensory areas of the brain interfere with the ability to successfully self-massage areas of the back and limbs?

   a. The largest sensory and motor awareness is in these areas

   b. The distribution of sensory and motor function to the hands is too small to stimulate sensation

   c. The distribution of sensory and motor function is larger to the hands than to the back and limbs

   d. The back and limbs have a predominance of sensory distribution over the motor distribution of the hands

112. A client is experiencing lingering anxiety from a minor auto accident 4 hours ago. What difference between the nervous system and the endocrine system would explain this condition?

   a. The nervous system is short acting and the endocrine system is long acting

   b. The endocrine system is short acting and the nervous system is long acting

   c. The nervous system transports hormones more consistently through blood and tissues

   d. Neurotransmitters have a long duration of effect and hormones are short acting

 Answers are on page 295.

113. *A 38-year-old female client describes symptoms of constipation, increased edema, sensitivity to cold, muscle and joint pain, and hair loss. She indicates that there is an increase in stress in her life; she is tired and seems unable to cope as effectively as before. She had a general physical examination within the last 6 months but no specific tests were done. Based on these symptoms, which condition might suggest a need for referral?*

    a. Exophthalmos
    b. Hypothyroidism
    c. Hyperthyroidism
    d. Hypocalcemic tetany

114. *A type 2 diabetic wishes to become a client for therapeutic massage. The physician is supportive. Which of the following statements is most accurate as a basic understanding of type 2 diabetes?*

    a. There is a disruption of insulin production from the islet cells of the pituitary gland
    b. Insulin is a powerful diuretic, so increased edema is a warning sign of diabetic coma
    c. Insulin is released when levels of blood sugar, amino acids, and fatty acids rise
    d. Glucagon facilitates the ability of insulin to transport glucose across the cell membrane

115. *If an intervertebral disk rupture occurs, what is the possible outcome?*

    a. Narrowed disk space due to leakage of the nucleus pulposus
    b. Narrowed intervertebral space due to rupture of the fontanelle
    c. Impingement of the nerve from pressure exerted by the sella turcica
    d. Increased space in the foramen impinging on the spinal cord

116. *A female client, age 67, has a history of smoking. This could indicate caution for compressive force used during massage for which reason?*

    a. Osteonecrosis
    b. Osteomyelitis
    c. Osteochondritis dissecans
    d. Osteoporosis

117. *A client complains of fatigue and muscle soreness after attempting to push a car that was stuck. Which of the follow best describes this action?*

    a. No movement was produced, so static force was generated
    b. Dynamic force was used since the car did not move
    c. Static force produced movement and energy expenditure
    d. Since the car did not move, little energy was expended

118. *A client was a sprinter in high school track and was very effective during short and quick runs. Now 10 years later the client is complaining of lacking the endurance to run 5 miles as part of a fitness program. The client is in good physical condition with no apparent reason for the difficulties. Which of the following offers the most plausible explanation for the client's condition?*

    a. The person has an abundance of slow twitch fibers in relationship to fast twitch fibers
    b. The person has an increased ability to manage oxygen debt
    c. The person's legs have a genetic tendency toward a makeup of more white anaerobic fibers
    d. The person has increased slow twitch fibers in the postural muscles

119. *Two clients describe accidents in which the muscles of their upper thigh were cut and now healed. Client A has a mobile scar with near normal function. Client B has tissue rigidity and reduced movement. What is the most plausible explanation?*

    a. Client A limited exercise and kept the area tightly wrapped during the healing process
    b. Client B had more satellite cell activity during healing, causing increased scar tissue
    c. Client A exercised during healing to stimulate satellite cells
    d. Client B experienced increased circulation and reduced adhesions

 Answers are on page 295.

120. *A massage practitioner notices that a client's skin has a yellowish gold color. This would be an indication of _____.*

   a. Cyanosis
   b. Anemia
   c. Fever
   d. Jaundice

121. *A massage professional identifies a few small lumps in the axillary area of a female client. What might be a pathologic concern?*

   a. Basal cell carcinoma
   b. Candidiasis
   c. Psoriasis
   d. Fibrocystic disease

122. *A client has a history of heart attack and has reduced blood flow to the heart. Which of the following vessels is most involved?*

   a. Coronary
   b. Left external carotid
   c. Celiac
   d. Renal

123. *What is the first heart chamber to receive blood from the superior and inferior venae cavae?*

   a. Right ventricle
   b. Right atrium
   c. Left ventricle
   d. Left atrium

124. *A client complains of pooling of blood in the lower extremities. Which of the following circumstances would be a likely cause?*

   a. Increased walking
   b. Lying with the feet above the heart
   c. Standing still for extended periods
   d. Regular deep breathing

125. *During a general massage the massage practitioner notices that the dorsalis pedis pulse is weaker on the left. Where is the practitioner palpating?*

   a. Upper arm
   b. Wrist
   c. Knee
   d. Ankle

126. *After a 1-hour massage focused on relaxation, a client becomes dizzy when sitting up. What is the likely cause?*

   a. Stimulation of baroreceptors
   b. Increase of sympathetic stimulation
   c. Pulse rate of 65 beats per minute
   d. Decrease in parasympathetic tone

127. *The immune function of mucus results because _____.*

   a. It is sticky
   b. It creates inflammation
   c. Of phagocytosis
   d. It washes pathogens from the body

128. *A client is immune suppressed. The physician has provided approval for massage. What would be the best massage treatment plan?*

   a. General massage with specific use of stimulation techniques to encourage sympathetic dominance
   b. General massage with a focus on aggressive lymphatic drainage
   c. General massage with active stretching to encourage parasympathetic dominance
   d. General massage to support nonspecific homeostatic regulation and restorative sleep

129. *Joint function is a combined relationship between _____.*

   a. Bones and landmarks
   b. Stability and mobility
   c. Articulations and diarthroses
   d. Synovial fluid and pathologic range of motion

Answers are on page 295.

130. A client has been participating in a stretching program for over a year. Initially the program was very helpful, but during the last 3 months the program has become more aggressive and the client is complaining of joint pain. Which alteration in connective tissue may explain what has occurred?

   a. The client has experienced a rupture in the connective tissue structures and has developed lax ligaments
   b. The client has exceeded the limits of the elastic range of the tissue, consistently deformed the tissue in the plastic range, and developed lax ligaments
   c. An avulsion failure of connective tissue has occurred, creating a decrease in mobility
   d. The tissue has become dehydrated, increasing creep tendency and contributing to stability provided by muscle contraction

131. A client has been diagnosed with a hypermobile knee joint. Which of the following would be part of an appropriate treatment plan?

   a. Extend the elastic range of connective tissue structures by altering the plastic range
   b. Elongate the plastic component of connective tissue in the direction of the shortening
   c. Restore pliability
   d. Manage muscle contraction around the joint using standard massage methods

132. A client complains of pain in the region of the low back and buttocks. Which dermatome nerve distribution might indicate where the nerve impingement is located?

   a. C-7
   b. T-2
   c. C-6
   d. L-2

133. The sensory receptors most affected by deep compression and slow gliding strokes are _____.

   a. Pacinian corpuscles
   b. Root hair plexuses
   c. Merkel's disks
   d. Ruffini's end organs

134. A client reports being prone to headaches from being in bright light. Bright light has only been a problem in the last few weeks. The client also reports an increase in workload. What might be the function of the ANS that could be responsible for the sensitivity to light?

   a. Parasympathetic dilation of the pupil
   b. Sympathetic dilation of the pupil
   c. Parasympathetic contraction of the pupil
   d. Sympathetic contraction of the pupil

135. A client reports having herpes zoster and is experiencing pain. Which of the following would be the best massage approach?

   a. A full-body 1-hour massage with attention to universal precautions that uses tapotement, active joint movement, and fractioning methods
   b. A full-body massage lasting 1_ hours that avoids the area of the rash and that actively engages the client in muscle energy lengthening and stretching
   c. A seated massage that lasts for 15 minutes
   d. A full-body, 1-hour massage that avoids the area of the rash with attention to universal precautions and a focus toward relaxation

136. Which of the following would most often be considered the fulcrum?

   a. Quadriceps muscles
   b. Radius
   c. Deltoid ligament
   d. Glenohumeral joint

137. During normal gait in the adult, the lumbar rotation is countered by a cervical spine rotation in the opposite direction for what reason?

   a. To keep the eyes on a level plane and the head oriented forward with the trunk
   b. To maintain the same-side counterbalance action of the arms and legs
   c. To coordinate the lever action of the elbows with the knees
   d. To activate the second-class lever system of the lift of the heel when moving onto the toes

 Answers are on page 295.

138. *An individual was running up stairs carrying a heavy briefcase in the left hand. Later that day the person felt increased tension in the left biceps muscle. Two days later, during a regular massage session, the client describes weakness and heaviness in one leg when walking up stairs or a hill. If normal gait reflexes are functioning, where would assessment likely find an inhibited muscle pattern?*

    a. Right arm extensors
    b. Left hip flexors
    c. Right hip flexors
    d. Left hip extensors

139. *Which of the following aspects of the gait cycle would result in most concentric contraction of the plantar flexors?*

    a. Heel strike
    b. Mid-stance
    c. Toe-off preswing
    d. Mid-swing

140. *A massage professional positions the client's body to assess the strength of the hip flexors. Which is the correct position for the hand applying resistance?*

    a. Near the hip
    b. At the ankle
    c. At the distal end of the femur
    d. On the tibia

141. *The prefix meaning against or opposite is _____.*

    a. Circum-
    b. Caud-
    c. Contra-
    d. Brach-

142. *The use of abbreviations in charting _____.*

    a. Is universally understood
    b. Is more time consuming
    c. Requires a deciphering key
    d. Clearly communicates information

143. *The cutaneous/visceral reflexes are correlated with which Chinese medicine concept?*

    a. Essential substances
    b. Pernicious influences
    c. Organ systems
    d. Five elements

144. *The common relationship between yin/yang, the five element theory, and Ayurvedic dosha is _____.*

    a. Entrainment
    b. Somatic
    c. Homeostasis
    d. Etiology

145. *Which of the following represent principles of movement?*

    a. Pitta
    b. Vata
    c. Kapha
    d. Ether

146. *A sensor mechanism, integration/control center, and effector mechanism are all part of a _____.*

    a. Stress response
    b. Postisometric relaxation
    c. Stimulus response
    d. Feedback loop

147. *Massage is part of a feedback loop in the _____.*

    a. Controlled condition
    b. Control center
    c. Response
    d. Stress stimulus

148. *Biologic rhythms are maintained by _____.*

    a. Circadian patterns
    b. Ultradian patterns
    c. Negative feedback
    d. Positive feedback

 Answers are on page 295.

149. *Relaxed mood states are experienced by people when _____.*

   a. Biologic rhythms are entrained to sympathetic patterns
   b. Biologic rhythms are oscillated independently
   c. Biologic rhythms are entrained to the chakra system
   d. Biologic rhythms are entrained to parasympathetic patterns

150. *Relaxation methods that focus on breathing produce entrainment because _____.*

   a. Cortisol increases during parasympathetic response.
   b. Respiration rate is a major biologic oscillator
   c. Sympathetic mechanisms are generated
   d. Baroreceptors are inhibited

151. *A disease with a vague onset that develops slowly and remains active for a long period of time is considered _____.*

   a. Acute
   b. Communicable
   c. Chronic
   d. Idiopathic

152. *Systemic inflammatory responses and fibromyalgia are _____.*

   a. Indicated for massage that causes inflammation
   b. Indicated for massage that involves extensive stretching and pulling techniques
   c. Contraindicated for massage that causes inflammation
   d. Contraindicated for massage only in the area of the joints

153. *Pathogenic disease-causing organisms include _____.*

   a. Dirt, sweat, and grime
   b. Paint, tar, and dust
   c. Viruses, bacteria, and fungi
   d. Smoking, drinking, and washing

154. *A client's low back pain returns within 3 hours of receiving massage. What organ may be the cause of referred back pain?*

   a. Bladder
   b. Kidney
   c. Stomach
   d. Gallbladder

155. *Massage used as a pain management strategy is a form of _____.*

   a. Stimulus-induced analgesia
   b. Acupuncture
   c. Dermatomal inhibition
   d. Prostaglandin stimulation

156. *Problem-oriented medical records including SOAP require that _____.*

   a. The qualified goals and the outcome of the massage be noted on the record
   b. The facts, possibilities, logical consequences of cause and effect, and impact on people be noted on the record
   c. The results of palpation assessment but not the client history be recorded
   d. Only the interventions be noted on the record

157. *The most important area in terms of determining future intervention procedures based on results is _____.*

   a. S: subjective—what the client states
   b. O: objective—what was observed from assessment and examination
   c. A: analysis—what worked/did not work
   d. P: plan—what client wants to work on and what needs to be done during the next session

158. *An individual response to professional therapeutic touch _____.*

   a. Is consistent with cultural influences
   b. Cannot be predetermined
   c. Is gender specific
   d. Depends on outcomes

                                    Answers are on page 295.

159. *Massage, the word, is derived from all the following languages **except** _____:*

    a. English
    b. French
    c. Arabic
    d. Greek

160. *The three primary ways pathogens are spread are person-to-person contact, environmental contact, and _____.*

    a. Handwashing
    b. Universal precautions
    c. Shoes
    d. Opportunistic invasion

161. *What is the massage trend that developed in 1991 that supported acceptance for the benefits of massage?*

    a. Increase in valid research
    b. Deregulation of massage education
    c. Decrease in influential women in the profession
    d. Resistance to integrating massage into traditional health care settings

162. *A client seems nervous and unwilling to provide information during the history-taking process. The massage therapist is becoming impatient. What is lacking?*

    a. Rapport between client and practitioner
    b. Prior information from the physician
    c. State-dependent memory status
    d. Proper clinical reasoning skills

163. *When are data collected during the assessment process interpreted as to patterns of dysfunction and methods of massage application?*

    a. As the history taking progresses
    b. During the physical assessment
    c. As the information is charted in the subjective section
    d. After the data have been collected and analyzed

164. *During the initial greeting, a client seems generally healthy and in good spirits; however, when the client is speaking the breathing pattern seems strained. What assessment process is being used?*

    a. Palpation
    b. Physical assessment
    c. Interviewing
    d. Observation

165. *A massage practitioner asks a client the following question, "Please explain to me how you would like to feel after the massage." What is correct about this communication?*

    a. The massage practitioner used an open-ended question
    b. The massage practitioner directed the response to reduce rapport
    c. The practitioner was formulating a response during listening to the answer
    d. A closed-ended interview was used to effectively use time

166. *A massage practitioner carefully listens to a client during the interview portion of the assessment process and then proceeds to the physical assessment. What communication step was forgotten?*

    a. Open-ended questions and analysis
    b. Charting and treatment plan development
    c. Summarizing and restating information
    d. Using understandable language

167. *A vacationing client will only have one massage from the massage practitioner. Which is the appropriate assessment process?*

    a. Subjective history taking for possible referral combined with a physical assessment for symmetry and gait assessment for optimal movement patterns
    b. Palpation assessment of soft tissues to identify treatment areas
    c. Subjective and objective assessment for contraindications
    d. Interviewing for client's quantitative goals

 Answers are on page 295.

168. During postural assessment the massage professional observes that the client's shoulder girdle is rotated to the left. Which of the following histories is most likely to be the cause?

    a. The client regularly reaches to the left when answering the phone
    b. The client often wears boots when riding horses
    c. The client does weight-bearing exercise with machines three times a week
    d. The client wears tight clothing

169. A regular client has a grade 2 left ankle sprain and is using a crutch to maintain balance when walking. During assessment of posture, the massage therapist notices an elevated right shoulder. What is happening to cause this?

    a. The client is closing an open kinetic chain pattern
    b. The muscles of the right lower leg are inhibited
    c. The symmetrical stance is enhanced
    d. The body is displaying compensation patterns

170. When one is observing for symmetry, which of the following is correct?

    a. The shoulders should evenly roll forward, leveling the clavicles
    b. The circumference of the muscle mass in the legs should be similar
    c. The ribs should be fixed more on the left and springy on the right
    d. The patella should be pointed more medially

171. Which of the following is part of a normal gait pattern?

    a. The arms swing freely opposite the leg swing
    b. The knee is maintained in the "screw-home" mechanism
    c. The toes contact the floor first and then roll to the heel
    d. During push-off the foot is dorsiflexed

172. In which area would additional study be required when working with any population with special needs?

    a. Massage methods
    b. Special situations
    c. Psychology
    d. Relaxation methods

173. An adult male client has many surgical scars on his chest and abdomen. History indicates that the client had surgical intervention as a child to repair congenital malformations. The client enjoys massage on the limbs and back in the prone position but appears distant and unsettled when turned to the supine position. What is the most logical explanation for this response?

    a. An abusive family history
    b. Reenactment
    c. Dissociation
    d. Integration

174. A college football player is seeking massage as part of a healing program for an injured knee that required surgical intervention. The athletic trainer is supervising the massage. The massage consists of general full-body massage that addresses any developing compensation caused by the gait change while the knee is healing. Specific applications of kneading and myofascial release are being used to maintain pliability in the soft tissue of the upper and lower leg. What type of massage is being performed?

    a. Postevent massage
    b. Recovery massage
    c. Remedial massage
    d. Rehabilitation massage

175. In which of the following circumstances would breast massage be most appropriate?

    a. General massage
    b. Adjunct to breast cancer treatment
    c. Scar tissue management
    d. Examination for lumps

176. *In which of the following circumstances would massage without supervision by a health care professional best benefit children?*

    a. Growing pains
    b. Anxiety disorder
    c. Touch sensitivity
    d. Attention deficient disorder

177. *A massage professional has been working with a client who has chronic pain syndrome. The massage helps when combined with physical therapy, judicious use of pain medications, and support group attendance. Improvement in the condition begins after six or seven massage sessions. After ten to twelve sessions the client misses three or four sessions, then returns for massage and indicates that she is right back where she started. She states that she doesn't feel like the situation will ever improve. What is the most logical explanation for this behavior?*

    a. State-dependent memory
    b. Decrease in hardiness
    c. Secondary gain
    d. Acute pain

178. *A client has been working on a project that required gripping a hammer for an extended period. Now the client is complaining of weakness when attempting to extend the wrist. Which of the following is the most likely explanation?*

    a. The flexor muscle group of the hand and wrist increased tone levels, resulting in inhibition of the extensor group of muscles in the forearm
    b. The flexor digitorum superficialis and profundus are weak from fatigue, so the wrist extensors have been facilitated
    c. The deep layer of the posterior wrist extensor group is antagonistic to the superficial layer of this same muscle group, resulting in weakness in the wrist extensors
    d. The flexor carpi ulnaris and the extensor carpi ulnaris are both in spasm, resulting in inhibition of the abductor pollicis longus

179. *While observing a client walk, the massage professional notices that the pelvis does not move evenly. The client complains of focused pain in the right sacral area. Which of the following is most correct?*

    a. Create a massage treatment plan describing specific treatment for sacroiliac dysfunction
    b. This information combined with other data may indicate the need for referral, with current massage focused on general nonspecific approaches
    c. Design a massage to lengthen the left leg to balance the pelvic rotation
    d. Immediately refer the client to a chiropractor for sacroiliac dysfunction

180. *A client is taking an anticoagulant. Which of the follow would be contraindicated?*

    a. Resting stoke
    b. Friction
    c. Muscle energy
    d. Rocking

181. *During the massage the massage professional notices a temperature difference in the tissue of the lumbar area. One area the size of a quarter is warmer than the surrounding area. Which type of assessment is being used?*

    a. Postural assessment
    b. Gait assessment
    c. Palpation
    d. Muscle testing

182. *Which of the following is the most effective way to assess for potential areas of muscle hyperactivity when the focus of the palpation is on the surface of the skin?*

    a. Compressing until the striations of the underlying muscles are felt
    b. Light fingertip stroking to assess for areas of dampness or drag
    c. Skin rolling to assess for any adherence of superficial fascia to the skin
    d. Moving the skin on top of the superficial fascia to locate areas of bind

 Answers are on page 295.

183. Sensory stimulation of massage causes a
chemical change in a neuron called _____.

   a. Action potential
   b. Refractory period
   c. Depolarization
   d. Saltatory conduction

184. Which of the following statements is most
correct?

   a. The body has no actual anatomic or
      physiologic functioning limits
   b. The body has only anatomic functioning
      limits
   c. The body has only physiologic functioning
      limits
   d. The body has anatomic and physiologic
      functioning limits

185. A person is clumsy and has a dull or foggy mind
in terms of understanding information and
making decisions. Which of the following
neurotransmitters may be involved?

   a. Norepinephrine
   b. Histamine
   c. Glutamate
   d. Dopamine

186. In relation to anatomy and physiology, the
phrase "structure and function" involves _____.

   a. Gross anatomy translates to regional
      anatomy
   b. Anatomy guides physiology and is modified
      by function
   c. Systemic physiology involves organizational
      anatomy
   d. Duality of wholeness represented in
      catabolism and anabolism

187. A client experienced an accident in which the
trunk was thrust into extension. Which of the
following structures might have been injured?

   a. Deltoid ligament
   b. Anterior longitudinal ligament
   c. ASIS
   d. Linea aspera

188. The process of homeostasis is a logical well-
coordinated pattern of balance. When balance is
disrupted patterns of dysfunction occur. Often
both homeostasis and disease begin at what level
of body organization?

   a. Chemical
   b. Cellular
   c. Tissue
   d. Organ

189. The concept of yang as compared to atomic
structure is _____.

   a. Nucleus
   b. Protons
   c. Electrons
   d. Neutrons

190. Which of the following is a description of
burning pain?

   a. Short-lived but intense and easily localized
   b. Constant but not well localized
   c. Slow to develop, lasts longer, and less
      accurately localized
   d. Blood supply to the muscle is occluded, and
      contraction causes pain

191. Which type of atomic bond holds together DNA?

   a. Ionic bond
   b. Covalent bond
   c. Polar covalent bond
   d. Catabolic bond

192. Feedback is an essential aspect of homeostasis
because of _____.

   a. Afferent discharge
   b. Effector response
   c. Information exchange
   d. Efferent signaling

                    Answers are on page 295.

193. If a client complains of pain in the buttocks and into the lateral side of the leg, which plexus is a potential site of nerve impingement?
    a. Cervical
    b. Brachial
    c. Lumbar
    d. Sacral

194. Pain, tingling, and numbness in the arm and hand may be the result from nerve damage in which plexus?
    a. Cervical
    b. Brachial
    c. Lumbar
    d. Sacral

195. A compressive massage method is applied to the belly of a muscle with the intent of reducing a muscle spasm brought on by a cramp. The receptors most affected are _____.
    a. Joint kinesthetic
    b. Golgi tendon organ
    c. Muscle spindles
    d. Meissner's corpuscles

196. Sacral plexus nerve impingement is indicated by _____.
    a. Gluteal pain, leg pain, genital pain, and foot pain
    b. Headaches, neck pain, and breathing difficulties
    c. Shoulder pain, chest pain, arm pain, wrist pain, and hand pain
    d. Low-back discomfort with a belt distribution of pain and with pain in lower abdomen, genitals, thigh, and medial lower leg

197. As slow deep effleurage is applied to the left upper thigh, the practitioner notices and the client describes a twitching of the muscles in the back of the opposite leg. What type of reflex has been stimulated?
    a. Stretch reflex
    b. Tendon reflex
    c. Ipsilateral reflex
    d. Contralateral reflex

198. A client complains of a sensation of thickness and stiffness in the myofascial structures of the body. Slow sustained stretching provides the most benefit. What is the most plausible reason for this effect?
    a. The neuromuscular unit is deprived of calcium, allowing the actin and myosin to disengage
    b. The viscous nature of connective tissue responds to this method by becoming more plastic
    c. The colloid connective tissue ground substance decreases water binding with these methods
    d. The compression against the capillaries increases blood flow

199. A client is complaining of pain when straightening the elbow. Palpation of the triceps at the musculotendinous junction indicates more tenderness at the insertion when the muscle is activated. What is the most likely reason for this?
    a. The insertion is the fixed attachment and would be more tender during movement.
    b. The insertion is the proximal attachment and is straining at the intermuscular septa
    c. The belly of the muscle located at the insertion is highly innervated
    d. The insertion is the more movable attachment so it would produce more tenderness upon motion

200. A client unexpectedly lifted a box that was much too heavy. Now the client is experiencing residual weakness in the biceps and brachialis muscles and tension in the triceps muscle group. Which of the following reflexes best explains this situation?
    a. Stretch reflex
    b. Tendon reflex
    c. Withdrawal reflex
    d. Crossed extensor reflex

    Answers are on page 295.

Practice Test Two

1. Which of the following is a violation of confidentiality?

   a. Maintaining client records in a secure location
   b. Asking the client questions about work environment
   c. Approaching and speaking to a client in a restaurant
   d. Speaking to a client's chiropractor with appropriate releases

2. *A client complains of pain in the tibia. The client completed a marathon 24 hours before the massage session. What contraindication to massage may account for the pain?*

   a. Stress fracture
   b. Compound fracture
   c. Dislocation
   d. Whiplash

3. *A massage professional has been working with a particular client for 12 months. Recently the client has been experiencing increasing difficulties with the family communications. The biggest problem is stress and tension between son and father. Discussions during massage are centered around solving this problem. Which of the following best describes this situation?*

   a. Massage professional is having difficulty maintaining informed consent
   b. Scope of practice violations, particularly with psychology, are occurring
   c. The client should be referred for either acupuncture or chiropractic
   d. The client is engaged in countertransference

4. *Research indicates that massage increases the body's availability of the following neurotransmitters—norepinephrine, serotonin, and dopamine. Which central nervous system disorder would be most benefited by massage?*

   a. Stroke
   b. Cerebral palsy
   c. Depression
   d. Schizophrenia

5. *During massage, pain that is not related to specific symptoms radiates around the ear. This indicates excessive pressure on which nerve?*

   a. Greater auricular
   b. Thoracodorsal
   c. Medial cutaneous
   d. Pudendal

6. *Which of the following receptors is most likely to adapt and cease responding to the sustained compression during massage on one specific area of the body?*

   a. Meissner's corpuscles
   b. Thermal receptors
   c. Type II cutaneous mechanoreceptors
   d. Nociceptors

7. *A client is complaining of a recent inability to sleep and a feeling of agitation and reports concern over a change in management systems at work. The physician diagnosis was exogenous anxiety. Which of the following treatment plans is most appropriate?*

   a. Mild exercise program, therapeutic massage, and a medication such as imipramine to control symptoms
   b. A hypoventilation syndrome management program including massage and chiropractic manipulation
   c. A mild exercise program, cognitive behavioral therapy, short-term use of diazepam, and relaxation massage
   d. Therapeutic massage, meditation, increase in caffeine consumption, and bed rest

8. *A client who is a marathon runner developed an inflammatory condition of the knee. As part of the treatment process, the client received an injection of corticosteroid into the area of the knee. The client wishes to have a deep massage of the area to reduce the pain. Why is this not appropriate?*

   a. The massage could decrease the inflammatory response and concentrate the medication at the injection site
   b. Deep massage increases the potential for localized inflammation and would disturb the action of the corticosteroid injection
   c. Deep massage would increase the tension of the muscles, causing instability, and inflammation would decrease
   d. Corticosteroids reduce inflammation and increase tissue repair; since massage increases the tendency for tissue repair, excessive scarring could result

9. *A client is experiencing pain on palpation of many points along the kidney meridian. Which element of the five elements contains the kidney meridian?*

   a. Fire
   b. Water
   c. Wood
   d. Earth

10. *A client has just experienced a job shift change from days to nights and is having difficulty adjusting the sleep pattern. The client indicates feeling disconnected and out of sorts. Which endocrine gland might initially be affected and which massage approach would be most beneficial?*

    a. Pineal gland; a massage that focuses on sympathetic stimulations with active participation by the client
    b. Adrenal glands; a massage that generates localized inflammatory areas, such as is found with direct pressure and friction on trigger points
    c. Thymus gland; a massage that uses sufficient pressure but pain-free compression and rhythmic gliding methods to support parasympathetic dominance
    d. Pineal gland; a massage that uses sufficient pressure but pain-free compression and rhythmic gliding methods to support parasympathetic dominance

11. *A young male client is experiencing a growth spurt. He complains that the bones in his legs ache. What is responsible for this phenomenon?*

    a. Increased testosterone promotes long bone growth
    b. Increased estrogen promotes long bone growth
    c. Decreased estrogen supports long bone growth
    d. Decreased testosterone promotes long bone growth

12. *A client complains of pain in the lower back. Observation indicates an excessive lumbar curve. This is called _____.*

    a. Scoliosis
    b. Kyphosis
    c. Lordosis
    d. Talipes

 Answers are on page 296.

13. A client is complaining of a feeling of shortening and pulling in the area of the low back and sacroiliac joints. Assessment indicates decreased pliability in the connective tissue structures in this area. Which of the following massage applications is most appropriate to achieve an increase in short-term mobility without compromising stability or creating a remodeling process of the tissue?

   a. Application of massage methods that slowly introduce creep, increasing pliability at the plastic range of the tissue
   b. Application of therapeutic inflammation coupled with stretching to exceed the plastic range of the tissue
   c. Application of elongation stretching to breach the plastic range of the tissue, creating inflammation to restore an appropriate creep pattern
   d. Application of abrupt bending of the connective tissue to support the increase in ligament laxity, thereby increasing mobility

14. We now know that biochemicals are responsible for most problems in behavior, mood, and perception of stress and pain. Which of the following is an example of this type of problem?

   a. Anxiety
   b. Obstructive sleep apnea
   c. Eczema
   d. Farsightedness

15. A client is experiencing spasms in the left thigh flexor muscles. An attempt to muscle test the area could result in a cramp. The massage professional remembers that activation of the gait reflexes can either facilitate or inhibit muscle contraction. Which group of muscles would the massage professional have the client contract in order to inhibit the left thigh flexors?

   a. Left arm flexors
   b. Right arm flexors
   c. Left arm extensors
   d. Right thigh extensors

16. A client is experiencing muscle spasms and reduced mobility around a shoulder joint that has a history of dislocation. Which of the following applications of massage would be best in assisting this client?

   a. Increase the plastic range of the ligament structures and stretched tense muscles
   b. Use friction on tendons and ligaments, then incorporate a stretching program to increase flexibility
   c. Reduce muscle spasms to the point that mobility is supported but stability is not compromised
   d. Use massage methods and stretching to eliminate muscle spasms

17. A massage practitioner has obtained required licenses for her business location. The type of business set up was a sole proprietorship with a DBA. She has her business checking account and tax plan developed with an attorney. She also contacted a local insurance agent for appropriate insurance. She is a member of a professional organization that supplies professional liability insurance. She has a marketing plan and client practitioner agreements. What did she forget?

   a. Retirement investment plan
   b. Zoning approval
   c. Salary structure
   d. Business plan

18. A client has a history of a broken wrist. The wrist was in a cast for an extended period of time because bone repair was slower than normal. The client is now experiencing a decrease in range of motion of the wrist. What might be the cause?

   a. Hypomobility due to contracture
   b. Hypomobility due to reduced muscle tension
   c. Hypermobility due to increased muscle tension
   d. Hypomobility due to increased anatomic range of motion

 Answers are on page 296.

19. During assessment the massage professional realizes that a client has extremely mobile joints. Which muscle functions would seem to be impaired?

    a. Produce movement
    b. Generate heat
    c. Maintain posture
    d. Stabilize joints

20. A client is complaining of tender areas in the postural muscles along the spine. Assessment indicates a series of trigger points in these muscles. The massage professional must determine how much compressive force to apply to the trigger points and how long to hold the contraction. Which of the following will affect this decision?

    a. These muscles contain more slow twitch red fiber that are fatigue resistant
    b. These muscles are prone to oxygen debt
    c. These muscles have an abundance of fast twitch and intermediate fibers
    d. These muscles require a maximal stimulus in order to respond to treatment

21. A client with fibromyalgia has been referred from the physician for massage. A treatment plan has been requested for approval before treatment begins. Which of the following would be the best approach?

    a. General massage with active assisted joint movement and stretching
    b. General massage with friction methods to active tender points
    c. Localized massage to the feet and ischemic compression to active trigger points
    d. General massage to support restorative sleep and symptomatic pain management

22. A client experienced an auto accident 4 years ago that resulted in a bulging disk at L-4. The injury has since healed with minimal difficulties. During assessment, palpation indicates a moderate decrease in pliability of the lumbar dorsal fascia and mild shortening in the lumbar muscles. Forward flexion and rotation of the lumbar area are mildly impaired. Massage was focused to reduce the muscle shortening in the lumbar area and increase connective tissue pliability. Immediately after the massage the client reported increased mobility but within 15 minutes began to complain of lower back pain. What is the most likely explanation for this occurrence?

    a. A shift of the condition from second-degree functional stress to first-degree functional tension
    b. Increase in stability around the past injury
    c. Decrease in mobility in the area around the past injury
    d. Destabilization of resourceful compensation in lumbar area around past injury

23. A client complains of joint pain in the knee and assessment indicates hypermobility with pain on passive movement. Which of the following would be the most appropriate treatment plan?

    a. General massage to the body with specific muscle energy work and lengthening of the extensors and flexors of the knee
    b. General massage with regional contraindications to the knee area and referral for more appropriate diagnosis of possible capsular dysfunction
    c. Referral for diagnosis prior to any massage
    d. General massage with attention to friction methods at the joint capsule

24. A client is experiencing an upper chest breathing pattern. Which of the following muscle(s) may test as short and too strong from this type of breathing?

    a. Diaphragm
    b. Suprahyoids
    c. Scalenes
    d. Infraspinalis

 Answers are on page 296.

25. A client complains of pain and tension in the lower back more to the left side. Physical assessment indicates that the pelvis is elevated on the left as compared to the right. The client also indicates difficulty raising the left arm over the head. Which of the following muscles may be involved?

    a. Psoas
    b. Rectus abdominis
    c. Latissimus dorsi
    d. Semispinalis

26. If the scapula remains fixed and immobile, what would result at the glenohumeral joint?

    a. Range of motion would be limited
    b. Internal and external rotation would be enhanced
    c. Flexion would be unaffected
    d. Horizontal abduction would be the only limitation

27. Which of the following functions of the integumentary system is supported by maintaining sanitary procedures?

    a. Protecting against water loss
    b. Detecting sensory stimuli
    c. Preventing entry of bacteria and viruses
    d. Excreting sweat and salts

28. Which of the following heart valves controls the flow of blood from the ventricles into the aorta?

    a. Atrioventricular
    b. Mitral
    c. Tricuspid
    d. Semilunar

29. When one feels confident with commitment, control, and challenge in life, one is _____.

    a. Coping well
    b. Using behavior modification
    c. Functioning from an external locus of control
    d. Reliant on defense mechanisms

30. A client is quite shy and modest. Which of the following draping methods would be the best choice?

    a. Contoured draping with towels
    b. Partial body towel draping
    c. Full body sheet and towel draping
    d. Sheet draping with no towels

31. Which of the following would be an indication for referral?

    a. A radial pulse of 85 beats per minute
    b. A femoral pulse of 55 beats per minute
    c. A carotid pulse of 70 beats per minute
    d. A dorsalis pedis pulse of 52 beats per minute

32. A massage professional has been working 12-hour days, 6 days a week, for 2 years. She is seeing 40 clients per week. Lately she finds herself tired and out of sorts. She does not attempt to rebook clients who cancel. What is the most logical explanation for her behavior?

    a. Motivation
    b. Coping mechanisms
    c. Burnout
    d. Infection

33. In polarity theory, how many major body currents exist?

    a. Two
    b. Three
    c. Five
    d. Seven

34. What is the water temperature for a neutral bath?

    a. 65 to 92 degrees
    b. 98 to 104 degrees
    c. 92 to 98 degrees
    d. 56 to 65 degrees

                    Answers are on page 296.

35. A client has had surgery for varicose veins in the legs. Which vein was removed?

    a. Azygous
    b. Brachiocephalic
    c. Hepatic
    d. Saphenous

36. Characteristics of life involve _____.

    a. Physiology
    b. Yin
    c. Anatomy
    d. Tissue

37. Which of the following is a temporary deficiency or diminished supply of blood to a tissue?

    a. Aneurysm
    b. Embolus
    c. Blockage of a vessel
    d. Ischemia

38. Both lymphatic ducts empty lymph fluid into the _____.

    a. Mediastinal nodes
    b. Subclavian veins
    c. Mesenteric artery
    d. Cisterna chyli

39. Massage that provides a pumping compression to the foot encourages lymphatic flow because _____.

    a. The palmar plexus is stimulated
    b. The parotid nodes are drained
    c. The plantar plexus is stimulated
    d. The mammary plexus is stimulated

40. A person had the measles as a child and is no longer susceptible. This is called _____.

    a. Nonspecific immunity
    b. Immune deficiency
    c. Specific immunity
    d. Phagocytosis

41. Which of the following is correct in application of trigger point therapy?

    a. 15-minute application in combination with lengthening and stretching
    b. 45-minute application with hydrotherapy cold applications
    c. Limiting application to active trigger points only
    d. Using pressure methods first and limiting lengthening

42. A client has been experiencing ongoing work and family stress and cannot seem to recover from an upper respiratory infection. What is the most logical cause?

    a. Ongoing stress increases natural killer cells
    b. Ongoing stress supports the development of autoimmune disease
    c. Ongoing stress suppresses T-cell activity
    d. Decrease in cortisol suppresses the immune system

43. A client is having difficulty being comfortable with the touch of draping material during the massage. He says that he cannot get used to the scratchy feeling. The client may be displaying a reduced ability of sensory receptors to _____.

    a. Send impulses
    b. Adapt to sensation
    c. Remain monosynaptic
    d. Initiate reciprocal inhibition

44. Myofascial methods are most specifically focused on change in the _____.

    a. Motor point
    b. Lymph nodes
    c. Gait control mechanism
    d. Ground substance

                    Answers are on page 296.

45. *A client with a diagnosis of asthma is referred for massage. What would be the most likely benefits of massage?*

   a. Activation of the sympathetic nervous system would support bronchoconstriction
   b. Reduction in anxiety and increased mobility of the ribs
   c. Stimulation of the client's ability to inhale but inhibition of excessive exhalation
   d. Increase in tone of respiratory muscles, supporting effective exhalation

46. *A client has severely limited all dietary fat. Which of the following might occur?*

   a. Inability to digest protein
   b. Difficulty with hormone production
   c. Interference with the absorption of water-soluble vitamins
   d. Decreased conversion of galactose

47. *Massage in Ayurvedic theory concentrates on _____.*

   a. Manipulation of the doshas
   b. Tapping, rubbing, and squeezing points called kapha
   c. Movement of fluid along the vata centers
   d. Tapping, rubbing, and squeezing points on the body called marmas

48. *Of the following, which is contagious?*

   a. Appendicitis
   b. Hepatitis
   c. Reflux esophagitis
   d. Irritable bowel syndrome

49. *Appropriate massage for the colon _____.*

   a. Begins at the ascending colon, ends at the rectum, and moves toward the cecum
   b. Begins at the sigmoid colon and ends at the cecum, with directional flow toward the rectum
   c. Begins at the rectum and ends at the cecum, with a directional flow toward the cecum
   d. Begins at the splenic flexure and ends at the hepatic flexure, with directional flow toward the sigmoid colon

50. *Erectile tissue is able to become firmer because _____.*

   a. This tissue engorges with blood
   b. Muscles contract, stiffening the tissue
   c. The tissue absorbs water from the lymph
   d. Smooth muscles encircle the tissue, acting as a sphincter

51. *The alkaline nature of semen is to _____.*

   a. Stimulate orgasm
   b. Counteract the acid nature of vaginal fluid
   c. Thin the protective coating of the ovum
   d. Lubricate the ejaculatory duct

52. *During strength muscle testing, both the flexors and the extensors of the elbow seem equally strong. Why is this a dysfunctional pattern?*

   a. Gait patterns should inhibit the flexors
   b. Flexors should be about 25% stronger than extensors
   c. Extensors should be 30% stronger than adductors
   d. Postural muscles are inhibited by gait reflexes

53. *A massage client does not provide effective feedback about the amount of pressure requested for massage. The client asks for very deep pressure. As the massage professional you keep asking if the pressure is causing pain and the client says no. It seems that any deeper pressure may cause bruising and other tissue damage. This client may be exhibiting _____.*

   a. Counterirritation
   b. Reduced influence of beta-endorphins
   c. High pain tolerance
   d. Hyperstimulation analgesia

54. *A 56-year old male client complains of difficulty voiding urine. What would be the most likely diagnosis from his physician?*

   a. Endometriosis
   b. *Trichomonas* vaginitis
   c. Bartholin cyst
   d. Benign prostatic hypertrophy

                    Answers are on page 296.

55. *A client is getting ready to play a tournament tennis game in 60 minutes. She wants to increase circulation and prepare her muscles for the game. Which of the following treatment plans in the best option?*

   a. Long gliding strokes from distal to proximal focused toward the heart combined with rocking. Duration of the massage—45 minutes.
   b. Broad-based compression to the soft tissue of the limbs generally focused from proximal to distal combined with shaking and tapotement. Duration of the massage—20 minutes.
   c. Full-body massage with muscle energy methods and lengthening. Duration of the massage—45 minutes.
   d. Compression, superficial myofascial release, and trigger point work focused on the limbs combined with passive joint movement and shaking. Duration of the massage—15 minutes.

56. *A client is experiencing weakness and exhaustion; impaired concentration, memory, and performance; disturbed sleep; and emotional sweating. A complete physical has ruled out any existing pathology. Stress is indicated as a probable cause. Which of the following treatment plans would best reverse the stress response?*

   a. Massage to promote lymphatic drainage and stimulate arterial circulation
   b. Massage to support proper breathing function and reverse hyperventilation syndrome
   c. Massage to reduce scar tissue and prevent adhesions
   d. Massage to stimulate increase in heart rate and blood pressure

57. *A massage professional needs an understanding of disease processes. This study of disease processes is called _____.*

   a. Pathogenesis
   b. Pathology
   c. Epidemiology
   d. Pharmacology

58. *Which of the following meridians is located on the lateral side of the body beginning at the ear and ending at the toes?*

   a. Pericardium
   b. Bladder
   c. Liver
   d. Gallbladder

59. *A massage therapist feels restless on days off and finds it more difficult to sleep. What is the most logical reason for this phenomenon?*

   a. Providing massage usually promotes a parasympathetic response in both the client and the practitioner; on days when no massage is performed, the practitioner does not stimulate relaxation responses as effectively
   b. Providing massage is fatiguing; on days off the massage practitioner has more energy
   c. Providing massage interferes with natural entrainment responses, and on days off the practitioner is more in tune with biorhythms
   d. Providing massage increases adrenaline and other stimulating hormones and neurotransmitters; when this occurs, hyperventilation syndrome is common, resulting in restlessness and sleep disturbances

60. *A middle-aged client is reluctant to work with a 22-year-old massage therapist. This is an example of _____.*

   a. Gender issues
   b. Genetic predisposition
   c. Age issues
   d. Body sensitivity

61. *Which of the following are forms of touch technique?*

   a. Socially stereotyped touch
   b. Mechanical touch
   c. Inadvertent touch
   d. Ritualized touch

                                    Answers are on page 296.

62. *The practice of acupuncture involves _____.*

    a. The stimulation of specific points along the body, usually by the insertion of tiny, solid needles

    b. The stimulation of specific points along the body, usually by the pressing of the thumb into the point

    c. The stimulation of broad points along the body, usually by accomplishing a series of ever-deepening compressive strokes

    d. Using counterirritation, such as scraping, cutting, or burning of skin, to relieve pain

63. *In Shiatsu the points are called _____.*

    a. Hara

    b. Meridians

    c. Jitsu

    d. Tsubo

64. *A massage professional does not regularly drape all clients in a modest and professional manner. Which of the following best describes this conduct?*

    a. The massage professional practices a dual role

    b. The massage professional has breached a standard of practice

    c. The massage professional is involved in misuse of the scope of practice

    d. The massage professional needs additional training in draping

65. *Ayurvedic theory classifies physiologic functions by _____.*

    a. Elements

    b. Visceral function

    c. Feedback

    d. Doshas

66. *A massage professional has been asked to work with a support group for persons with cerebral palsy. The therapist is well trained and has 7 years of experience but is uncomfortable with people with disabilities, especially if communication is problematic. Which of the following is grounds for refusal on the part of the massage professional?*

    a. Lack of skills

    b. Lack of peer support

    c. Inability to serve without bias

    d. Only wishes to work with females

67. *RICE applications for first aid are appropriate for _____.*

    a. Primary care of abrasion

    b. Grade 2 and 3 sprains and strains

    c. Neural injury

    d. Shock

68. Which of the following is the best example of transference?

    a. A massage professional is biased toward a client due to political beliefs

    b. A massage professional is receiving small gifts from a client expressing affection

    c. A massage professional asks a client to attend a meeting about a nutritional product with him

    d. A client is angry with the massage professional for being late for the last three appointments

69. *Massage sensations travel on which spinal cord tracts?*

    a. Sensory ascending tracts

    b. Motor descending tracts

    c. Corticospinal tracts

    d. Lateral reticulospinal tracts

70. *In Ayurvedic theory, bones, flesh, skin, and nerves belong to which element?*

    a. Ether

    b. Air

    c. Earth

    d. Water

                    Answers are on page 296.

71. *Record keeping for clients involves _____.*

    a. Charting each session of the ongoing process
    b. Having the client fill out a general information packet
    c. Written record of intake procedures, informed consent, needs assessments, recording of each session, and release of information
    d. Filing each piece of information received from physicians, insurance companies, or payments received from clients

72. *Allergy is a condition of _____.*

    a. Immune system suppression
    b. Lack of T-cell activity
    c. Overactive immune response
    d. Immune deficiency

73. *Which of the following would be recorded in the objective data section of a SOAP note?*

    a. Client states she has interrupted sleep
    b. Client is currently taking melatonin
    c. Observation and palpation indicate upper chest breathing
    d. Client wishes to have weekly appointments

74. *The purpose of valid research in massage is to _____.*

    a. Generate more questions about massage
    b. Objectively research the physiologic process
    c. Subjectively research the massage process
    d. Justify massage as an art

75. *A massage practitioner notices that he becomes a bit aloof if he gets behind and is late for scheduled massage sessions. This is a/n _____.*

    a. Denial measure
    b. Defensive measure
    c. Exhaustion phase response
    d. Lack of purpose

76. *Wellness usually involves simplification of lifestyle to reduce demands. A stressful outcome of this process is often _____.*

    a. Hyperventilation syndrome
    b. Financial stability
    c. Dealing with loss and letting go
    d. Increased social support

77. *In relationship to ancient chakra theory, if someone is concerned with not having enough money to pay bills, surviving a job change, and staying focused learning a new computer skill, which endocrine gland is likely to be affected?*

    a. Pituitary
    b. Thyroid
    c. Adrenal
    d. Pineal

78. *Which methods directly affect (stimulate) the nervous system?*

    a. Mechanical methods
    b. Circulatory methods
    c. Reflexive methods
    d. Connective tissue methods

79. *Massage can increase a person's fine motor movements such as handwriting. Which neurotransmitter is influenced?*

    a. Serotonin
    b. Oxytocin
    c. Dopamine
    d. Growth hormone

80. *Massage has been demonstrated to reduce some people's craving for food and/or reduce hunger. Which neurotransmitter is responsible?*

    a. Epinephrine
    b. Serotonin
    c. Dopamine
    d. Norepinephrine

 Answers are on page 296.

81. If I wanted my employees to be more attentive, I would do massage for _____.

   a. 5 minutes
   b. 45 minutes
   c. 15 minutes
   d. 60 minutes

82. An objective measurement of connective tissue shortening in the lumbar area would be _____.

   a. Measuring a skin fold by lifting the tissue
   b. Placing the client in the prone position and having her lift her chest off the table into extension
   c. Measurements of hot and cold skin temperature
   d. Palpation of adjacent pulse points for evenness

83. In the human body, what initiates entrainment?

   a. Digestive glands
   b. Autonomic nerves
   c. Brain
   d. Biologic oscillators

84. The Arndt-Shultz law states: Weak stimuli activate physiologic processes; very strong stimuli inhibit them. What are the implications for massage?

   a. Massage is a strong sensory stimulation
   b. Techniques have to be intense to produce responses
   c. It is difficult to figure out if a pain originates from a joint or surrounding tissue
   d. To encourage a specific response, use gentler methods; to shut off the response, use deeper methods

85. The best way to increase arterial flow circulation enhancement during massage is _____.

   a. A 50-minute massage using effleurage but not heavy pressure
   b. A 45-minute compressive massage against the arteries proximal to the heart and moving in a distal direction
   c. A 50-minute massage using short pumping effleurage and gliding toward the heart
   d. A 30-minute massage emphasizing gliding strokes to passive/active joint movement distal to proximal

86. During the interview process, a client continues to grab the tissue at the back of the neck and pull it. What is the most logical explanation for this gesture?

   a. Nerve entrapment
   b. Joint compression
   c. Trigger point
   d. Connective tissue shortening

87. The triple heater meridian location corresponds with which nerve?

   a. Ulnar nerve
   b. Tibial nerve
   c. Sciatic nerve
   d. Lateral plantar nerve

88. A client enters the massage room complaining of a bad back from working at the computer. There are no stated contraindications. This is a stage one dysfunction. The client wants to reverse the condition. Which approach is the best process?

   a. Refer to low-back specialist
   b. Therapeutic change
   c. Condition management
   d. Palliative care

89. Which of the following people may require only palliative care from a massage therapist?

   a. An athlete with a sprained ankle
   b. A 48-year-old female with a broken arm
   c. A man with terminal cancer
   d. A pregnant woman in the first trimester

                    Answers are on page 296.

90. *Pathology can be best defined as _____.*

    a. The in-between state of not healthy but not sick
    b. Anatomic and physiologic functioning limits
    c. The study of disease
    d. Processes of inflammatory tissue repair

91. *The root word pneum(o)- means _____.*

    a. Vein
    b. Lung or gas
    c. Chest
    d. Breathing

92. *Homeostasis can be defined as _____.*

    a. The process of counterbalancing a defect in body structure or function
    b. A group of signs and symptoms
    c. The relative constancy of the body's internal environment
    d. The subjective abnormalities felt by the patient

93. *What is it called when new cells are similar to those that they replace?*

    a. Egestion
    b. Fibrosis
    c. Inflammation
    d. Regeneration

94. *Inflammation that persists beyond beneficial healing is considered an inflammatory disease. This chronic form of inflammation may be helped with what form of massage?*

    a. Extensive application of deep transverse friction
    b. Light surface stroking
    c. Controlled use of friction, stretching, and pulling
    d. Brisk beating and pounding

95. *The generally accepted definition of chronic pain is _____.*

    a. A symptom of a disease condition or a temporary aspect of medical treatment
    b. Pain frequently experienced by clients who have had a limb removed
    c. Pain that persists or recurs for indefinite periods, usually longer than 6 months
    d. Pain that often subsides with or without therapy

96. *If a client is experiencing pain in a surface area away from the stimulated organ, this is termed _____.*

    a. Muscle pain
    b. Referred pain
    c. Deep pain
    d. Acute pain

97. *Cold applications of hydrotherapy to reduce swelling are called _____.*

    a. Analgesic
    b. Antipyretic
    c. Antispasmodic
    d. Antiedemic

98. *Neck pain on the right side can be indicative of referred pain from what organs?*

    a. Appendix and kidney
    b. Colon and bladder
    c. Heart and lungs
    d. Liver and gallbladder

99. *Relaxed ordered entrainment is produced by massage in response to _____.*

    a. The practitioner's direct application of methods
    b. The practitioner's calm presence and rhythmic application
    c. The practitioner's emotional state
    d. The practitioner's specific choice of methods that address the chakra system

          Answers are on page 296.

100. *Intervention is different for managing acute versus chronic pain. Acute pain is managed* _____.

   a. With inhibitory methods
   b. Using aggressive rehabilitation approach
   c. Less invasively and focused to support current healing process
   d. By compression on a nerve in a bony structure

101. *What is the major reason that massage practitioners need to be aware of endangerment sites?*

   a. These are soft areas that are unable to tolerate any pressure or movement
   b. They may be a sign of a life-threatening disorder
   c. The remaining proximal portions of sensory nerves are exposed here
   d. These areas are not well protected by muscle or connective tissue, so deep sustained pressure could damage vessels, nerves, or other structures

102. *Predisposing conditions that may make the development of disease more likely by the client than by another person are called* _____.

   a. Metastasis
   b. Pathology
   c. Signs
   d. Risk factors

103. *A massage professional is troubled over a client's responses during the last four massage sessions. There is nothing specific about the client's behavior, but something has changed in the client's response to the massage. What could be helpful to the massage professional?*

   a. Credentialing review with certification
   b. Managing intimacy issues
   c. Changing body language
   d. Decision making with peer support

104. *A doctor referral is indicated if the* _____.

   a. Client has mild edema in the lower legs after a plane flight
   b. Client complains about care at the local outpatient client
   c. Client bruises easily
   d. Client is beginning a new medication

105. *A group of simple parasitic organisms that are similar to plants but have no chlorophyll and live on skin or mucous membranes are* _____.

   a. Viruses
   b. Fungi
   c. Bacteria
   d. Protozoa

106. *Pathogens are spread by three main routes. Which of those below is one of these?*

   a. Opportunistic invasion
   b. Clean uniform
   c. Intact skin
   d. Aseptic technique

107. *Pressurized steam bath would be an example of what common aseptic technique?*

   a. Isolation
   b. Sterilization
   c. Disinfections
   d. Universal precautions

108. *Acquired immunodeficiency syndrome is defined as* _____.

   a. An inflammatory process caused by a virus
   b. Human immunodeficiency virus
   c. A group of clinical symptoms caused by a dysfunction in the body's immune system
   d. A disease contracted by casual contact such as shaking hands or sharing bathroom facilities

                    Answers are on page 296.

109. *Universal precautions are defined as _____.*

   a. Emergency care given to all ill or injured persons before medical help arrives
   b. Procedures developed by the CDC to prevent the spread of contagious disease
   c. The process by which all microorganisms are destroyed
   d. The process by which pathogens are destroyed

110. *What is the most efficient standing position?*

   a. Symmetrical
   b. Wide stance (shoulder length apart)
   c. Asymmetrical
   d. Lead foot with the pressure on it

111. *Most massage applications use a force generated _____.*

   a. Downward
   b. Forward
   c. Downward and forward
   d. Forward and across

112. *A massage professional is feeling strain in the shoulders and arms after doing four massage sessions. Which of the following is the most logical reason?*

   a. The massage professional is using muscle strength in the arms to exert force
   b. The massage professional is standing in an asymmetrical stance
   c. The client is positioned for best mechanical advantage
   d. The massage professional is effectively leaning up hill

113. *A massage professional is complaining of pain in the wrist and near the elbow. Which of the following is an appropriate corrective action?*

   a. Maintain the hands in a clenched fist to promote stability
   b. Increase the movement of the stroke at the shoulder joint
   c. Relax the hand and fingers during massage
   d. Shift the compressive force to the fingers and thumb

114. *Observation of a fellow massage practitioner indicates that the shoulder girdle is aligned with the pelvic girdle, the pressure-bearing arm opposite the weight-bearing leg, the fingers relaxed, the head up, the back straight, the elbows bent, and the stance asymmetrical. Which of these areas needs correction?*

   a. Elbows
   b. Stance
   c. Back position
   d. Shoulder position

115. *In the earth element, if the stomach is yang, then what is yin?*

   a. Spleen
   b. Bladder
   c. Liver
   d. Triple heater

116. *Increasing levels of pressure are achieved by _____.*

   a. Moving closer to the massage table
   b. Moving away from the massage table
   c. Standing on the toes
   d. Shifting the weight-bearing foot to the front

117. *A client is particularly concerned with safely and is afraid of falling. Of the following massage equipment, which would make the client most comfortable?*

   a. Mat
   b. Stationary table
   c. Portable table
   d. Chair

118. *To maintain sanitary practice, draping material must be _____.*

   a. Laundered in hot soapy water with a disinfectant such as bleach
   b. Sterilized and heat pressed
   c. Professionally laundered
   d. Warm, large enough to cover the client, and different colors

                    Answers are on page 296.

119. The purpose of lubricant is _____.
    a. To moisturize the skin
    b. To reduce friction on the skin
    c. To transport nutrients
    d. Counterirritation

120. A client comes to you complaining of an aching pain just under the ribs right of the midline, under the right scapula, and in the right neck and shoulder area. The pain has been occurring on a more frequent basis and is now almost constant. The referred pain pattern might indicate problems with what organ?
    a. Bladder
    b. Kidney
    c. Stomach
    d. Gallbladder

121. A massage professional is preparing an orientation process for a new client. The professional has developed the following checklist: Show client massage area, where to change and hang clothes, massage table draping and positioning, how to get on and off the massage table, music choices, and restrooms. Explain charts and equipment, lubricant types, sanitary procedures, and privacy methods. What did the massage professional forget?
    a. To explain the general idea of massage flow
    b. To provide a centering meditation with the client
    c. To provide education on self-help
    d. To introduce the client to products for sale

122. The history-taking interview provides data for which part of the SOAP note charting process?
    a. Subjective data
    b. Objective data
    c. Analysis
    d. Plan

123. Which of the following is contraindicated for application of deep sustained compression?
    a. Lymph nodes
    b. Trigger points
    c. Dermatomes
    d. Ground substance

124. A massage practitioner uses massage manipulations in a brisk and specific way. Which of the following client goals is best served by this approach?
    a. Decreased alertness
    b. Increased parasympathetic response
    c. Decreased sensory awareness
    d. Increased alertness

125. Many ancient healing practices were developed based on _____.
    a. Measurement of concrete functions
    b. Experiential observation
    c. Scientific methods
    d. Meridian system

126. A massage client is unhappy with the massage. The main complaint is a feeling of choppiness and lack of continuity. Which of the following qualities of touch is most responsible?
    a. Depth of pressure
    b. Drag
    c. Rhythm
    d. Direction

127. Which of the following methods has as its primary effect a lifting of the tissue away from underlying structures?
    a. Compression
    b. Petrissage
    c. Gliding
    d. Vibration

128. In which pathologic process would massage be most beneficial in assisting in the movement of body fluids?
    a. Upper motor neuron injury
    b. Lower motor neuron injury
    c. Aneurysm
    d. Chorea

 Answers are on page 296.

129. *A couple has experienced difficulties conceiving a third child. The doctors can find no reason for the difficulties. The male is a regular client. He asks if massage could be of help. The answer is yes. Which of the following justification statements is most logical?*

    a. Massage can assist in the success of sexual intercourse by encouraging adrenaline secretion
    b. Massage can increase the rate of ovulation by stimulating the hypothalamus to secrete follicle-stimulating hormone
    c. Massage can encourage more efficient homeostatic mechanism in the body, promoting general health, including fertility
    d. Massage can increase the levels of testosterone, prolactin, and progesterone, promoting ovulation

130. *When the outcome for the massage is to produce parasympathetic dominance, which combination of methods would be the best choice?*

    a. Gliding, rocking, and passive joint movement
    b. Compression, shaking, and friction
    c. Active joint movement, reciprocal inhibition, and rocking
    d. Tapotement, compression, and vibration

131. *The main therapeutic focus of polarity therapy is to _____.*

    a. Balance the tridosha system
    b. Restore balance in the yin/yang system
    c. Remove structural imbalance
    d. Locate blocked energy and release it

132. *Many benefits of massage are a result of _____.*

    a. Nonspecific stress stimulus that encourages feedback response to more optimum function
    b. Precise application of selected stimulus creating positive feedback
    c. Positive feedback response to return function to homeostasis
    d. Afferent transmission to the sensory mechanism with the disrupted homeostasis reduced by the control center

133. *A client requests that tapotement be used at the end of the massage to stimulate the nervous system. Which is the best choice for the face?*

    a. Hacking
    b. Cupping
    c. Tapping
    d. Slapping

134. *Which of the following is produced voluntarily?*

    a. Joint play
    b. Arthrokinematic movement
    c. Osteokinematic movement
    d. Joint end-feel

135. *A client's muscles cramp when the massage professional attempts to use postisometric relaxation to lengthen a shortened group of muscles. Which of the following methods would be a better choice to lengthen the muscle group?*

    a. Skin rolling
    b. Active resistive joint movement
    c. Reciprocal inhibition
    d. Stretching

136. *Which method is being described? Isolate the target muscle in passive contraction. Have the client contract the antagonist group. Have the client relax and then lengthen the target muscles.*

    a. Postisometric relaxation
    b. Reciprocal inhibition
    c. Contract-relax antagonist contract
    d. Pulsed muscle energy

137. *A client is ticklish, particularly on the chest. Which method would be the best choice to use in this area?*

    a. Compression over the client's own hand
    b. Friction
    c. Gentle effleurage
    d. Fingertip compression

 Answers are on page 296.

138. Which method is beneficial to use on the hands and feet to stimulate lymphatic movement?

    a. Superficial effleurage
    b. Skin rolling
    c. Vibration
    d. Pumping compression

139. A client has a lot of body hair on his back. During the first massage lubricant was used. At the return visit the client requests that lubricant not be used on his body where there are large amounts of hair. Which method could be used?

    a. Gliding
    b. Kneading
    c. Compression
    d. Petrissage

140. A client likes to have the back massaged and asks that most of the massage time be focused on the back. The client continues to complain that the massage is not very effective in reducing back pain. What explanation can be given to the client?

    a. The soft tissue of the back often is tight because of extensive pulling and shortening of the tissues in the chest; massage of the chest may help
    b. Massage to the back limits blood flow, so the soft tissues remain in contracture
    c. Massage on the extremities would be better to reduce the pain in this area since the mechanical effect is more concentrated
    d. The connective tissues of the back respond best to reflexive measures, and using a more generalized approach would provide relief

141. If pathology occurs because of a state of "too much" or "not enough," then health would occur because of _____.

    a. Increased immune activity
    b. Decreased sympathetic arousal response
    c. Effective feedback and adaptive capacity
    d. Tolerance and hardiness

142. A client notices that the massage office is clean, neat, and efficient and that licenses and certifications are posted on the wall. The client is impressed with the massage practitioner's abilities in _____.

    a. Applications of massage
    b. Communication skills
    c. Marketing
    d. Management

143. During the history interview a client reports that she almost fell down stairs but caught herself and was able to regain her balance. What type of reflex action was required to accomplish this?

    a. Monosynaptic
    b. Polysynaptic
    c. Patellar
    d. Pacinian

144. Which of the following is of most concern when massaging the face?

    a. Proximity to mucous membranes and transmission of pathogens
    b. The skin of the face is thin
    c. Facial muscles are weak
    d. Compression damages underlying cranial sutures

145. Which of the following body areas requires special attention to draping?

    a. Hand
    b. Leg
    c. Chest
    d. Shoulder

146. A client arrives late for a massage appointment. The remaining time is 30 minutes. The goal for the session is general relaxation. Which combination is the best choice to achieve desired outcomes in the allotted time?

    a. Back, gluteals, and hips
    b. Face, hands, and feet
    c. Hands, arms, and back
    d. Face, neck, and shoulders

Answers are on page 296.

147. When one is using passive joint movement as an assessment method, which of the following is being identified?

    a. End feel
    b. Viscosity
    c. Vessels
    d. Pilomotor reflex

148. A client is experiencing pain on palpation of many points along the kidney meridian. Which element of the five elements contains the kidney meridian?

    a. Fire
    b. Water
    c. Wood
    d. Earth

149. Bilateral assessment of the dorsalis pedis pulse would provide information about _____.

    a. Respiration
    b. Abdominal viscera
    c. Lymph nodes
    d. Arterial circulation

150. During palpation assessment, the massage practitioner wishes to assess for the status of the acupuncture meridians. Where would the practitioner focus the assessment?

    a. Tendons at the proximal attachment
    b. Ligament of synovial joints
    c. Grooves in fascial sheaths
    d. Myotomes

151. Which of the following is **incorrect** when using strength muscle testing?

    a. Isolate muscles and position attachments as close together as is comfortable
    b. Use a force sufficient to recruit a full response of the tested muscles and the surrounding muscles
    c. Use a slow and even counterpressure to pull or push the muscle out of the isolated position
    d. Compare muscle tests bilaterally for symmetry

152. A client is complaining of weakness and heaviness in the muscles that flex the left thigh. During muscle testing, the muscle group is found to be inhibited. Based on gait patterns, which of the following muscle groups should also be inhibited?

    a. Right arm flexors
    b. Left arm flexors
    c. Right thigh flexors
    d. Left thigh extensors

153. If the area between C-7 and T-12 is pulled forward, making the chest concave, with a right rotation pattern making the right shoulder more forward than the left, where are the shortened soft tissues?

    a. Anterior thorax on the right
    b. Right lumbar posterior
    c. Left thorax posterior
    d. Lower abdominal on the right

154. Which of the following is contraindicated for application of deep sustained compression?

    a. Lymph nodes
    b. Trigger points
    c. Dermatomes
    d. Ground substance

          Answers are on page 296.

155. A physician refers a client for massage for circulation enhancement to the limbs. The client complains of cold hands and feet. Assessment indicates decreased pliability of the tissues around the elbows and knees. Work-related activities require repetitive movement in these areas. The massage professional presents three main approaches for the physician to consider:
     1. General massage and rest
     2. General massage with connective tissue stretching in the restricted areas
     3. Compression focused specifically to the arteries to encourage circulation
     After considering all three options, the physician eliminates number 1 as too time consuming. Option 2 seems viable, but the client does not respond well to methods that may be painful. Option 3 seems too limited an approach to the massage professional. The decision is to begin with option 3 and expand to connective tissue methods when the client is able to tolerate them. Which part of this process best reflects brainstorming possibilities?

     a. Data collection
     b. Eliminations of options based on pros and cons
     c. Generating the options
     d. Assessment for more facts

156. A client experienced an episode of severe low back pain 3 years ago. The diagnosis was a compressed disk at L-4. The condition has stabilized and pain is experienced only occasionally. Assessment indicates shortened lumbar fascia, increased lateral flexion to the right, and a high shoulder on the right. The massage professional specifically addressed these areas and noted improvement following the massage. The next day the client called complaining that the low back was in spasm. What is the most logical reason for what happened?

     a. The phasic muscles were too weak to maintain posture
     b. The gait shifted so that there was a more normal heel strike
     c. Facilitated segments in the skeletal muscles went into spasm
     d. Resourceful compensation patterns were disturbed

157. When one is evaluating a treatment plan for successful client compliance, which of the following would provide the best information?

     a. Any referral information from the heath care provider
     b. Completing a comprehensive physical assessment
     c. Generating multiple treatment options
     d. Indications of enthusiasm for the plan by the client and any support system

158. Bodywork methods that focus on meridians and points fall into which category?

     a. Eastern and Oriental
     b. Reflex
     c. Energetic
     d. Structural

159. Which environment is the most difficult for maintaining professional boundaries?

     a. Public events
     b. Private office commercial building
     c. On-site residence
     d. Home office

160. Reflexology can be beneficial because _____.

     a. The complex structure of the foot is highly innervated and sensitive to changes in pressure and position, making it highly responsive to massage manipulation
     b. The flexor withdrawal mechanism of the foot is inhibited with pressure to the foot, and this inhibits neural activity in the dorsal horn of the spinal cord
     c. The specific mapped areas of reflex activity in the foot to organs have a direct relationship to visceral/cutaneous responses
     d. Stimulation of the zone therapy points on the bottom of the foot activates meridian energy movement in the chakra system

Answers are on page 296.

161. A client is experiencing pain with any activity involving external or lateral rotation of the right shoulder. Range of motion is limited to 40 degrees. This condition has been coming on gradually. Muscle testing indicates weakness when resistance is applied to move the shoulder from external rotation to internal rotation. There is shortening in the muscles of internal rotation. Which of the following would be the most logical treatment plan?

   a. Muscle energy methods to support lengthening of the infraspinatus and methods to increase tone in the subscapularis
   b. Deep massage to the rhomboids and stretching of the lumbar fascia
   c. Traction of the scapulothoracic junction
   d. Massage to reduce tension in the pectoralis major and latissimus dorsi with tapotement to increase tone in the infraspinatus and teres major

162. Why might massage be contraindicated for those with renal insufficiency?

   a. Massage causes increase in blood pressure
   b. Massage increases blood volume through the kidneys
   c. Massage spreads bacteria through the urinary system
   d. Massage increases the difficulty with incontinence

163. A client is experiencing pain on palpation of many points along the kidney meridian. Which element of the five elements contains the kidney meridian?

   a. Fire
   b. Water
   c. Wood
   d. Earth

164. In the five-element theory, what is the relationship of water to fire?

   a. Yin
   b. Yang
   c. Inhibiting
   d. Facilitating

165. Heat, redness, swelling, and pain are signs of _____.

   a. Cancer
   b. Degeneration
   c. Counterirritation
   d. Inflammation

166. A system of health and medicine developed in India is called _____.

   a. Prana
   b. Elements
   c. Polarity
   d. Ayurveda

167. Lung and diaphragm pain may be referred to which cutaneous area?

   a. Left side of the neck
   b. Right side of the chest
   c. Right side of the neck
   d. In the hip girdle area

168. A client complains of increased hunger and thirst, feels hot, and has been in a bad temper lately. Which of the Ayurvedic elements is out of balance?

   a. Earth
   b. Fire
   c. Water
   d. Ether

169. If an area of blocked energy is located, a simple polarity method is to _____.

   a. Place the left hand on the painful area and the right hand opposite the painful area
   b. Rub the area with specialized oil preparations
   c. Press into the area with the fire finger and hold
   d. Stimulate the corresponding marma

170. In polarity therapy, the heel of the foot is in a reflex relationship with the _____.

    a. Shoulders and chest
    b. Pelvis
    c. Head and brain
    d. Abdomen

171. An interesting similarity between the traditional chakra system and biologic oscillators is _____.

    a. Rhythm patterns
    b. Vibratory rate
    c. Shared location
    d. Size comparison

172. When one is considering the wellness components of balanced body, mind, and spirit, in which of the following intervention areas is massage most effective?

    a. Promoting exercise
    b. Restoration of an appropriate eating and sleep cycle
    c. Normalization of breathing mechanisms
    d. Promoting belief system changes

173. The law of facilitation states: When an impulse has passed through a certain set of neurons to the exclusion of others one time, it will tend to take the same course on a future occasion, and each time it travels this path the resistance will be smaller. What are the implications for massage?

    a. If a sensory receptor is activated, it will respond in a certain way
    b. Methods must override a sensation to produce a response
    c. The body likes sameness; after a pattern has been established, less stimulation is required to activate the response
    d. For a massage method to change a sensory perception, the intensity of the method must match and then exceed the existing sensation

174. A massage therapist is involved with developing a promotional campaign to increase his massage business since taking on a part-time massage employee. What is this called?

    a. Marketing
    b. Business plan
    c. Resume
    d. Management

175. Gross income minus expenses equals _____.

    a. Deductions
    b. Deposits
    c. Net income
    d. A draw

176. In which situation would you stay in the massage room and assist a client on and off the massage table?

    a. A client in the first trimester of pregnancy
    b. A 65-year-old male with diabetes
    c. An elderly female with high blood pressure
    d. An adolescent with a wrist cast

177. Trigger points are commonly located in _____.

    a. Ligaments
    b. Tendons
    c. The joint capsule
    d. Muscles

178. A client has increased internal rotation of the right shoulder. Which of the following is the best massage approach to reverse the condition?

    a. Frictioning and traction to the external rotators
    b. Muscle energy with lengthening and then stretching of the internal rotators
    c. Compression and tapotement to the internal rotators
    d. Stretching of the flexors and extensors with lengthening to the external rotators

Answers are on page 296.

179. The attachment of myosin to cross-bridges on actin requires _____.

    a. Calcium
    b. Maximal stimulus
    c. Endomysium
    d. Potassium

180. An adult male client has many surgical scars on his chest and abdomen. History indicates that the client had surgical intervention as a child to repair congenital malformations. The client enjoys massage on the limbs and back in the prone position but appears distant and unsettled when turned to the supine position. What is the most logical explanation for this response?

    a. An abusive family history
    b. Reenactment
    c. Dissociation
    d. Integration

181. A massage practitioner has been asked by a group of mental health professionals to begin working at a residential facility. She would need to be most concerned over which of the following?

    a. Types of mental health issues
    b. Obtaining informed consent
    c. Learning specific massage protocols for each condition
    d. Frequency and duration of the massage

182. The nervous system and the endocrine system reflect quantum properties because _____.

    a. Predictable physiologic outcomes are constant
    b. Feedback loops reliably affect outcomes
    c. Linear pathways of affect are constant
    d. Tendency for response is most accurate

183. Which aspect of bone structure provides the elastic quality of bone?

    a. Inorganic mineral
    b. Organic material
    c. Trabeculae
    d. Endoskeleton

184. Which of the following ancient healing systems most correlates with the endocrine system?

    a. Meridian system
    b. Five elements
    c. Doshas
    d. Chakra system

185. Massage therapy benefits conditions by encouraging the body through the phases involved in rehabilitation, restoration, and _____ of anatomic and physiologic function.

    a. Secretion
    b. Normalization
    c. Control
    d. Circulation

186. A client is experiencing a limitation in range of motion of the hip into abduction. Assessment indicates shortening and tension in the adductor group of muscles. Which of the following is the most likely source of the limited range of motion?

    a. Agonists
    b. Synergists
    c. Antagonists
    d. Fixators

187. Which of the following conditions is most likely to benefit directly from a nonspecific general massage session?

    a. Contusion
    b. Anterior compartment syndrome
    c. Muscle tension headache
    d. Spasticity

188. The external intercostal muscles create a vacuum in the thorax in which way?

    a. The upper ribs expand
    b. The ribs are pulled together
    c. The lower ribs are lifted up and out
    d. The diaphragm muscle arches upward

189. *Joints in which stability is reduced because of increased laxity of supportive ligaments will also have an increase in _____.*

   a. Joint play
   b. Hypomobility
   c. Muscle relaxation
   d. Plasma membrane

190. *A client requests an outcome from the massage session that includes a good night's sleep and less fidgeting. The massage session would then need to be designed to accomplish what?*

   a. Cranial sacral plexus inhibition
   b. Parasympathetic inhibition
   c. Sympathetic inhibition
   d. Sympathetic dominance

191. *Should there be an injury to the sternoclavicular joint that limits its range of motion, what other structure will be affected?*

   a. Radius
   b. Olecranon
   c. Scapula
   d. Deltoid ligament

192. *A client seeks massage after a diagnosis of neuralgia in the left leg. Which of the following would be a realistic therapeutic massage outcome?*

   a. Reduction of pain and regeneration
   b. Long-term symptom decrease
   c. Short-term pain management
   d. Short-term regeneration

193. *An elderly client with a history of slow tissue healing and gradual weight loss begins to stabilize her weight and increase her ability to heal skin abrasions after receiving a weekly massage for 3 months. Which of the following offers the most concrete explanation for this outcome?*

   a. Massage influences positive feedback mechanism to decrease adrenal output
   b. Massage supports hypothalamic release of growth hormone–releasing hormone
   c. Massage changes sleep patterns to increase dopamine influence
   d. Massage beneficially influences tissue transport systems of neurotransmitters from endocrine tissues

194. *A client sprained the joint in one of the fingers. What is going to be the most comfortable position for the joint and why?*

   a. The closed packed position because this is the most stable position of the joint
   b. The loose packed position so that movement can most easily occur
   c. The least packed position to accommodate swelling
   d. The closed packed position to accommodate increased synovial fluid

195. *The sympathetic chain ganglia are located in an area similar to the Back-shu points on which meridian?*

   a. Spleen
   b. Kidney
   c. Liver
   d. Bladder

196. *Neurotransmitters work in excitatory and inhibitory pairs. Which of the following would provide a balancing action for enkephalin?*

   a. Somatostatin
   b. Substance P
   c. Serotonin
   d. GABA

                      Answers are on page 296.

197. *During assessment you want the client to externally rotate the hip. What instructions would you give the client?*

    a. Please move your leg so that you cross it over the other leg at the ankles

    b. Please straighten your legs and turn the entire leg so that you point your toes toward each other

    c. Please straighten your legs and turn the entire leg so that you point your toes away from each other

    d. Please bring your knee toward your chest

198. *The massage method that most affects the inner ear balance mechanisms is _____.*

    a. Tapotement

    b. Compression

    c. Friction

    d. Rocking

199. *The purpose of therapeutic (feel good) pain during massage to manage undesirable pain is to stimulate which neurotransmitters?*

    a. Serotonin and endorphin

    b. Epinephrine and histamine

    c. Acetylcholine and dopamine

    d. Histamine and substance

200. *Muscle uses which of the following to produce mechanical energy to exert force?*

    a. Myoglobin

    b. Adenosine triphosphate

    c. Perimysium

    d. Cholecystokinin

                    Answers are on page 296.

B

Answer Key One

1. a	52. c	103. d	154. b
2. a	53. b	104. c	155. a
3. d	54. a	105. b	156. b
4. c	55. b	106. d	157. c
5. c	56. c	107. b	158. b
6. d	57. a	108. a	159. a
7. a	58. c	109. b	160. d
8. c	59. a	110. c	161. a
9. c	60. b	111. c	162. a
10. d	61. a	112. a	163. d
11. c	62. b	113. b	164. d
12. b	63. c	114. c	165. a
13. a	64. a	115. a	166. c
14. a	65. b	116. d	167. c
15. b	66. b	117. a	168. a
16. a	67. c	118. c	169. d
17. b	68. b	119. c	170. b
18. c	69. a	120. d	171. a
19. b	70. d	121. d	172. b
20. c	71. d	122. a	173. c
21. d	72. d	123. b	174. d
22. b	73. c	124. c	175. c
23. b	74. b	125. d	176. a
24. c	75. d	126. a	177. c
25. c	76. b	127. a	178. a
26. a	77. b	128. d	179. b
27. b	78. c	129. b	180. b
28. a	79. b	130. b	181. c
29. d	80. b	131. d	182. b
30. b	81. c	132. d	183. c
31. a	82. c	133. d	184. d
32. d	83. b	134. b	185. d
33. a	84. c	135. d	186. b
34. d	85. c	136. d	187. b
35. b	86. c	137. a	188. a
36. d	87. b	138. b	189. b
37. a	88. d	139. c	190. c
38. d	89. c	140. c	191. c
39. c	90. b	141. c	192. c
40. b	91. d	142. c	193. c
41. a	92. c	143. c	194. b
42. d	93. d	144. c	195. c
43. c	94. a	145. b	196. a
44. b	95. a	146. d	197. d
45. d	96. c	147. d	198. b
46. a	97. b	148. c	199. d
47. a	98. d	149. d	200. b
48. c	99. c	150. b	
49. b	100. c	151. c	
50. b	101. a	152. c	
51. b	102. c	153. c	

Answer Key Two

1. c	52. b	103. d	154. a
2. a	53. c	104. c	155. c
3. b	54. d	105. b	156. d
4. c	55. b	106. a	157. d
5. a	56. b	107. b	158. a
6. a	57. b	108. c	159. c
7. c	58. d	109. b	160. a
8. b	59. a	110. c	161. d
9. b	60. c	111. c	162. b
10. d	61. b	112. a	163. b
11. a	62. a	113. c	164. c
12. c	63. d	114. a	165. d
13. a	64. b	115. a	166. d
14. a	65. d	116. d	167. a
15. a	66. c	117. a	168. b
16. c	67. b	118. a	169. a
17. a	68. b	119. b	170. b
18. a	69. a	120. d	171. c
19. d	70. c	121. a	172. c
20. a	71. c	122. a	173. c
21. d	72. c	123. a	174. a
22. d	73. c	124. d	175. c
23. b	74. b	125. b	176. d
24. c	75. b	126. c	177. d
25. c	76. c	127. b	178. b
26. a	77. d	128. b	179. a
27. c	78. c	129. c	180. c
28. d	79. c	130. a	181. b
29. a	80. b	131. d	182. d
30. c	81. c	132. a	183. b
31. a	82. a	133. c	184. d
32. c	83. d	134. c	185. b
33. c	84. d	135. c	186. c
34. c	85. b	136. b	187. c
35. d	86. d	137. a	188. c
36. a	87. a	138. d	189. a
37. d	88. c	139. c	190. c
38. b	89. d	140. a	191. c
39. c	90. c	141. c	192. c
40. c	91. b	142. d	193. b
41. a	92. c	143. b	194. c
42. c	93. d	144. a	195. d
43. b	94. c	145. c	196. b
44. d	95. c	146. b	197. c
45. b	96. b	147. a	198. d
46. b	97. d	148. b	199. a
47. d	98. d	149. d	200. b
48. a	99. b	150. c	
49. b	100. c	151. b	
50. a	101. d	152. a	
51. b	102. d	153. a	